Radiation Oncology Clinical Fundamentals

John J. Cuaron • Lior Z. Braunstein
Editors

Radiation Oncology Clinical Fundamentals

Springer

Editors
John J. Cuaron
Department of Radiation Oncology
Memorial Sloan Kettering Cancer Center
New York, NY, USA

Lior Z. Braunstein
Department of Radiation Oncology
Memorial Sloan Kettering Cancer Center
New York, NY, USA

ISBN 978-3-031-77561-1 ISBN 978-3-031-77559-8 (eBook)
https://doi.org/10.1007/978-3-031-77559-8

This Springer imprint is published by the registered company Springer Nature Switzerland AG
The registered company address is: Gewerbestrasse 11, 6330 Cham, Switzerland

Preface

Radiation oncology stands at the forefront of modern medical practice, entwining over a century of technological advancement with the art of patient care. This handbook is crafted to be a practical and comprehensive guide for both seasoned clinicians and trainees, alike providing essential insights into the contemporary practice of radiation therapy. Our goal is to bridge the gap between the expansive literature in our field and its clinical application, providing a resource that is both informative and eminently practical.

As practitioners in the field, we vividly remember our own early careers, during which we often found ourselves seeking a resource that not only elaborated deeply on the principles of radiation therapy, but also provided a comprehensive synthesis of its practice. Despite the wealth of information available, we struggled to find a high-quality distillation that combined detailed, evidence-based knowledge with practical, real-world application. Further, while some texts and guides excel in defining the "what" and the "why" of radiation oncology principles, few include a detailed exploration of the "how." It is this unmet need that inspired us to create this handbook.

Recent decades have seen remarkable advances in radiation therapy. Innovations such as intensity-modulated radiation therapy (IMRT), image-guided radiation therapy (IGRT), and stereotactic body radiation therapy (SBRT) have allowed for unprecedented precision in targeting tumors and improvements in the sparing of adjacent tissues. The integration of advanced imaging modalities, such as positron emission tomography (PET) and magnetic resonance imaging (MRI), have further enabled the highly accurate delineation of target volumes and, most recently, real-time adaptation of exceedingly complex treatment plans.

The shift toward personalized medicine has also been a pivotal development in radiation oncology. Biomarkers and genetic profiling, bolstered by advancements in computational algorithms and artificial intelligence, now allow for treatments to be tailored to individual presentations, optimizing therapeutic efficacy while minimizing adverse effects.

Despite these advancements, the core principles of radiation oncology remain grounded in a deep understanding of radiation physics and cancer biology, and in a profound commitment to compassionate patient care. This handbook seeks to provide a balanced perspective, combining practical guidelines with the latest research and clinical evidence. It addresses major considerations in radiation oncology, including patient assessment, treatment planning, and delivery techniques.

Our hope is that this handbook will serve as the resource we wished for during our formative years—a trusted companion that offers practical advice, evidence-based recommendations, and a foundation for continuous learning.

We extend our heartfelt gratitude to the contributors and reviewers, whose expertise and dedication have made this handbook possible. Their collective wisdom and commitment to excellence are reflected in every chapter of this volume. We also acknowledge the patients, whose generosity of spirit and resilience inspire us daily to strive for better.

It is with great pleasure that we present this handbook on radiation oncology practice. We hope it represents a valuable resource in the practice of this most remarkable branch of medicine.

New York, NY, USA John J. Cuaron
New York, NY, USA Lior Z. Braunstein

Contents

CNS Radiation Therapy: Primary Brain Tumors, Brain Metastases, SRS, and Post-Op SBRT

1

Melissa R. Zinovoy, Kathryn Beal, Andrew R. Barsky, Yao Yu, and Luke R. G. Pike

CNS: Primary CNS Tumors

Glioblastoma and High-Grade Glioma

Chart Review/History of Present Illness (HPI)

- Clinical symptoms
- Risk factor assessment
- Physical Exam: performance status, incision check, neurologic exam
- Surgical Report: extent of resection
- Pathology review: MGMT promoter methylation status, IDH status
- Clinical trial review: particularly for unmethylated tumors
- Imaging: if rapid regrowth, consider re-resection
- Preoperative MRI with contrast
  - Fuse T1 post-contrast
- Post-operative MRI with contrast and perfusion
  - Fuse 3D slice T1 post-contrast and T2/FLAIR sequences
    Preferably within 7 days of simulation

M. R. Zinovoy (✉) · A. R. Barsky · Y. Yu · L. R. G. Pike
Department of Radiation Oncology, Memorial Sloan Kettering Cancer Center, New York, NY, USA
e-mail: remism@mskcc.org; barskya@mskcc.org; Yuy2@mskcc.org; PikeL@mskcc.org

K. Beal
Department of Radiation Oncology, Memorial Sloan Kettering Cancer Center, New York, NY, USA

Department of Radiation Oncology, New York-Presbyterian, New York, NY, USA
e-mail: kab4027@med.cornell.edu;

J. J. Cuaron, L. Z. Braunstein (eds.), *Radiation Oncology Clinical Fundamentals*,
https://doi.org/10.1007/978-3-031-77559-8_1

Simulation

- Three-point mask.
- IV contrast.
- Request fusion of above studies.
- RT to start approximately one month after surgery, but move up for clinical urgency, symptoms, and/or subtotal resection or after re-resection due to rapid tumor re-growth.

Dose/Contouring

- Dose
  - 60Gy in 30 fx for GBM [1], 59.4Gy in 33 for HGG
- Contouring
  - MSKCC preferred regimen:
    Volumes as per the EORTC (Stupp) approach:
    - GTV: Cavity plus enhancing disease on CT and MRI
    - CTV: GTV + 2 cm + expansion to include associated FLAIR
      - Adjust CTV for anatomical boundaries (bone, falx, optic structures, tentorium; allow crossing of the corpus callosum; can crop out of the brainstem if not involved)
    - PTV: CTV + 0.3–0.5 cm
  - RTOG alternative [2]
    Dose: 46 Gy/23 fx with boost to 60 Gy/30 fx
    Volumes
    - GTV1: T2/FLAIR abnormality on post-operative MRI scan.
    - CTV1: GTV1 + 2 cm
    - PTV1:CTV1 + 0.3–0.5 cm
    - GTV2 (Boost): Contrast-enhancing T1 abnormality post-op
    - CTV2: GTV + 2 cm
    - PTV2: CTV2 + 0.3–0.5 cm
  - Elderly/poor KPS alternative dosing:
    Dose:
    - 40 Gy/15 fractions [3]
      - Consider dose escalation to an EQD2 of 60Gy as a single course or via simultaneous integrated boost for select patients—52.5 Gy/15 fx [4]
    - Very poor KPS: 25–40 Gy/5 fractions (generally prefer 25Gy, although phase II data exist for 40Gy in 5 fx) [5, 7]

    Volumes:
    - CTV_40: (GTV + FLAIR signal) + 1 cm margin
    - CTV_52.5: GTV + 0–0.5 cm
      - GTV = Post-operative cavity and contrast-enhancing residual tumor
    - PTV: 0.3 cm
  - Gliomatosis/Multifocality or leptomeningeal disease:
    Treatment should be dictated by KPS, as prognosis is otherwise guarded in such cases, but options include:
    - Low KPS: see above, best supportive care
    - High KPS: 46 Gy/23 fx WBRT with boost to total of 60 Gy/30 fx with or without CSI

- Recurrence:
  - Dose:
    - 35 Gy/10 fx [6]
    - 30 Gy/5 fx
  - Volumes:
    - GTV: enhancing disease
    - CTV: 0 mm
    - PTV: 5 mm
  - Concurrent Avastin preferred in these cases [6]
  - If long disease-free interval or distant disease from the initial site
    - Consider more definitive dosing (e.g., 40.05–50.4Gy) and proton therapy

Image Guidance

- Daily KVs

Status Check

- Dexamethasone for symptoms only, with appropriate GI and PCP prophylaxis for extended courses
  - If ALC consistently <0.5 or on >2 mg of dexamethasone daily for at least 4 weeks
    - add Bactrim prophylaxis
  - Weekly CBC

Follow-Up

- 4 weeks post-RT
  - MRI Brain HGG with and without IV contrast with perfusion
    - Perfusion component important to differentiate tumor versus necrosis
  - Coordinate imaging with neuro-oncology

Low-Grade Gliomas

Chart Review/HPI

- Clinical Symptoms.
- Risk factor assessment [8]
  - Subtotal resection
  - Age >/= 40 yo
  - Tumor size >/= 4–6 cm
  - Tumor crosses midline
  - Refractory seizures
  - Presurgical neurologic symptoms from tumor
- Physical Exam: performance status, incision status, neurologic exam
- Surgical Report: extent of resection.
  - If there is rapid regrowth, consider re-resection.
- Pathology review: 1p19q deletion, IDH status
  - Discuss IDH mutant cases with neuro-oncology for consideration of IDH inhibitor versus radiation

- Clinical trial review
  - Particularly IDH-mutated tumors
- Treatment recommendations per ASTRO Clinical Practice Guidelines [8]
  - Oligodendroglioma, IDH-mutant, 1p/19 codeleted, or astrocytoma, IDH mutant

    G2
    - STR
      - Chemoradiation
    - GTR
      - If risk factors treat with chemoradiation
      - If no risk factors may surveil

Imaging

- Pre-operative MRI with contrast
  - Fuse T1 post-contrast and T2/FLAIR
- Post-operative MRI with contrast and perfusion
  - Preferably within two weeks of simulation
  - Fuse thin slice T1 post-contrast and T2/FLAIR sequences

Simulation

- Three-point mask
- No IV contrast
- Request fusion of above studies
- Ideally, schedule treatment within one month of surgery
  - Biopsy only or subtotal resection start as soon as possible

Contouring: [8]

- GTV: Enhancing disease on CT and MRI, resection cavity, and FLAIR changes
- CTV: GTV + 1.0 cm respecting anatomical boundaries
- PTV: CTV + 0.5 cm

Dose/Fractionation

- Grade 2 (54 Gy in 1.8 Gy fx)
- Grade 3 (59.4 Gy—60 Gy in 1.8–2.0 Gy fx)

Treatment

- IGRT: daily KVs

Status Check

- Dexamethasone management
  - If ALC consistently <0.5 or on >2 mg of dexamethasone daily for at least 4 weeks

    add Bactrim prophylaxis
  - Weekly CBCs

Follow-Up

- 4 weeks post-RT
  - MRI Brain HGG with and without IV contrast with perfusion
    Perfusion component important to differentiate tumor versus necrosis
  - Coordinate imaging with neuro-oncology

CNS: Brain Metastases

Whole-Brain Radiotherapy (WBRT)

History

- Clinical Symptoms
- Physical Exam: performance status, neurologic exam
- Neurosurgery consultation
  - pathologic confirmation
  - large tumors
  - symptomatic tumors
  - highly edematous tumors
- Pathology review: primary disease site

Indications

- Leptomeningeal carcinomatosis
- High intracranial burden of disease (e.g., >15 metastases, but no hard cutoff)
- Frequent or rapid recurrences following SRS
- High risk histology
  - Small cell lung cancer metastases patients [9]
  - Non-seminomatous germ cell tumors/germinoma

Imaging

- MRI with and without IV contrast

Simulation

- Three-point mask
- IV contrast
- IMRT/VMAT approach with hippocampal avoidance and memantine should be considered standard of care, with opposed laterals used for clinically symptomatic cases same-day or next-day start
  - Fuse thin slice T1 post-contrast and T2/FLAIR sequences for delineation of hippocampi and any nearby targets, obtained within 1 week of CT SIM

Dose/Fractionation/Fields

- Dose
  - 30 Gy/10 fx standard but 20Gy/5 fx acceptable alternative
- Volume:

  - WBRT: Inferior field border at C2/C3
  - Hippocampal-avoidance whole-brain radiation
    PTV = Brain +0.3 cm
    - Subtract bilateral hippocampi +0.5 cm (PRV-HA)

Modality

- Contraindications to HA-WBRT [10]
  - Leptomeningeal disease
  - Disease in the hippocampal-avoidance region (although unilateral sparing or partial sparing can be attempted with delineation of the target GTVs to be covered and ALARA to PRV-HA otherwise)
  - Urgent start required for symptoms

Additional

- Memantine
  - Goal:
    Prevention of cognitive dysfunction and improved quality of life [11]
  - Indication
    Expected survival >6 months
  - Dose: dose escalation with either short acting or long acting as per clinical trial (e.g., short acting starting at 5qd, then increasing to 5bid, 10qam, 5qpm, and then 10bid, total duration six months) [12]
  - Check creatinine prior to prescribing
  - Generally very well tolerated, but GI side effects are the most common (e.g., nausea)

Image Guidance

- WBRT
  - Daily kV
- HA-WBRT
  - Daily CBCT

Stereotactic Radiosurgery (SRS)

History

- Clinical Symptoms
- Physical Exam: performance status, neurologic exam
- Pathology review:
  - Primary disease site
  - Mutational burden
- Systemic therapy
  - Assess CNS penetrance
- Neurosurgery consultation
  - Pathologic confirmation

  - Large tumors
  - Symptomatic tumors
  - Highly edematous tumors
- Prior radiation record review

Indications

- Lower intracranial burden of disease
  - typically <15 metastases [13]
- First brain metastasis treatment
- Limited prior courses of SRS
- Select small cell lung cancer metastases patients [9]

Imaging

- MRI with and without IV contrast
  - 3D T1 post-sequence (1 mm slices) to be fused to 1 mm slice CT SIM
  - MRI must be acquired within 1 week of CT SIM, preferably less

Simulation

- Frameless rigid immobilization (e.g., CDR frame or Encompass, with Aquaplast mask).
- IV contrast
- Request fusion of above studies

Contouring

- GTV: Enhancing disease on both CT and MRI images
- PTV: GTV + 1 mm for uncertainty setup is standard; if uncertainty is greater, then consider 2 mm or re-SIM on a case-by-case basis (e.g., known rapid growth of disease)

Dose/Fractionation on Basis of Lesion PTV Diameter

- 0–2 cm: 21 Gy/1 fx
  - For clusters of lesions in which V12 (single fraction) or V18 (multi-fraction) will be larger and bleeding between lesions (e.g., with a total diameter > 2 cm), then have a low threshold to fractionate to the next dose level
- 2–3 cm: 27 Gy/3 fx (preferred) or 18Gy in 1 fx (alternative) [14]
- 3+ cm, any brainstem involvement, or for post-op cases: 30 Gy/5 fx (standard, with deviations from this to be justified otherwise)

Image Guidance

- Daily CBCT, match to bone but evaluate for shifts in gross anatomy (e.g., from hydrocephalus, bleeding, or cavity shifts at time of film approval)

Radiosurgery Steroid Premedication

- Dexamethasone
- Indications

  - Prophylaxis of acute edema, at physician discretion (e.g., from day 1 SRS, QD dosing of 6, 6, 4, 4, 2, 2)
  - Bulky or symptomatic tumors with significant mass effect/edema
- Contraindications:
  - Brittle diabetes
  - Immunotherapy (goal: keep dose <4 mg daily or not at all, if possible)
  - Volume overload (decompensated CHF)
- Consider Ativan usage as an anxiolytic or for seizure prophylaxis (temporal or motor strip lesions)
  - 0.5–1 mg Ativan 1–2 hours prior to SRS

Status Check

- Taper steroids, set up follow-up appointments

Follow-Up

- MRI with T1 3D post-contrast and perfusion sequences (e.g., MRI HGG + C + P) with clinic visit 1–3 days after this scan
  - First at 6–12 weeks post-treatment on the basis of risk
    (e.g., singleton brain metastasis s/p surgical resection may consider 10–12 weeks, while for a patient with >10 intact brain mets with untreated/indeterminate lesions, would suggest 6 weeks)
  - Every 2–3 months thereafter, with interval adjusted per clinical status

Post-Operative Stereotactic Body Radiation Therapy (SBRT)

History

- Clinical symptoms
- Physical exam: performance status, neurologic exam
  - Assess wound healing
- Pathology review:
  - Confirm primary disease site
  - Mutational burden
- Systemic therapy
  - Assess CNS penetrance
- Prior radiation record review

Imaging

- Preoperative MRI with and without contrast
  - Assess high-risk areas of contact with dura, large vessels/sinuses, and OARs
- Post-operative MRI with and without contrast
  - Fuse 3D T1 post-contrast and T2 imaging
  - Obtain ~7 to 10 days post-op, within 2–3 days of CT SIM

Simulation

- Five-point mask
- IV contrast
- Request fusion of above studies
- Timing
  - Treatment must be delivered within 1 month of surgery, preferably 1–3 weeks post-op with that time frame adjusted for clinical reasons. Immediate CT SIM is discouraged due to potential for cavity shifts between SIM and treatment and marginal misses.

Contouring

- Volumes [15]
  - GTV: any residual enhancing disease, surgical cavity, and tract
  - CTV: GTV + 1–2 mm, and further manually expanded along high-risk areas (e.g., dura in contact with tumor pre-treatment) an additional 3–5 mm
  - PTV: 1 mm standard with increase to 2 mm for rapidly growing disease or dynamic cavity, although re-SIM is preferred in the latter situation
- Multidisciplinary evaluation
  - Peer review of volumes with high-volume radiation oncologists
  - Review radiology reports and surgical notes in detail
  - Discuss case with radiologist, neurosurgeon

Dose/Fractionation

- 30 Gy/5 fx is the institutional standard
  - Alternative dosing:

    27Gy in 3 fx for small cavities (<3 cm PTV)—do not undercover CTV to achieve this

    25Gy in 5 fx or 30Gy in 10 fx for very large cavities, with the same approach to volumes

    Single fraction post-op SRS is *discouraged* on the basis of the exceedingly high failure rates seen in RCTs (as compared to WBRT)

    Consider SIB of 35Gy in 5 fx to gross disease in radioresistant histologies (e.g., GI, melanoma)

Treatment

- Treat 2–3 weeks post-operatively if cleared by neurosurgery
- IGRT: Daily CBCT as per above with careful review of bone alignment and check for cavity shifts

Status Check As per SRS guidelines above

Follow-Up As per SRS guidelines above

Leptomeningeal Carcinomatosis (LMD) [16]

Chart Review/HPI

- Clinical Symptoms
- Physical Exam: performance status
  - KPS, neurologic deficits, extent of systemic disease
- Pathology review
  - Non-small cell lung cancer and breast cancer
  - All other solid tumor histology
- Imaging review
- Multi-disciplinary discussion with neuro-oncology, medical oncology, and neurosurgery

Workup

- Mandatory for all patients:
  - MRI brain with 3D T1 post-sequences
  - MRI total spine with or without contracting
  - Lumbar puncture (if clinically safe, through either neuro-oncology or neuroradiology)

    Send: cytology, cell counts, glucose/protein, CTC (for tumor types expressing EpCAM), ctDNA (MSK IMPACT solid)

    Check anticoagulation status and time discontinuation prior to LP
  - CBC/Comp
  - Focused history and neurologic exam
  - Neuro-oncology referral
  - Recent systemic imaging
- Patients with leptomeningeal disease frequently may experience pressure-related symptoms due to hydrocephalus. These symptoms can require urgent palliation. Consider early referral to neurosurgery for shunt placement prior to RT in such cases.
- For suspected cases in patients with high KPS and limited extracranial disease, ***early*** referral to a proton radiation oncologist for consideration of proton craniospinal irradiation (pCSI) and obtain a "backup" CT SIM for possible VMAT CSI and/or WBRT.

Simulation

- WBRT to C2/C3 with three-point mask and focal spinal RT field as indicated per imaging and symptoms
- pCSI
  - Custom rigid immobilization
  - MRI fusions

Contouring

- pCSI
  - CTV entire brain, thecal sac, and proximal sacral nerve roots

- PTV typically 3–5 mm

Dose/Fractionation

- 30Gy/10 fractions

Image Guidance

- Daily Kvs

Treatment

- Best Supportive Care
  - Indications: major neurologic deficits, extensive systemic disease, and without good systemic therapies, poor KPS
- Whole brain radiation +/− focal spinal radiation for bulky or symptomatic disease
  - Indications: KPS < 60%, poor marrow reserves, urgent treatment required
- Proton Cranial Spinal Irradiation
  - Indications: KPS >60%, non-small cell lung cancer, and breast cancer; consider for other solid tumor histologies
  - Adequate bone marrow function
    - Hemoglobin >8 g/dl
    - ANC >1000/mm
    - Platelet >100,000/mm
- Memantine for all brain radiation

Follow-Up

- Every three months

Proton Therapy in Adult Brain Tumors

- Highly considered for:
  - Leptomeningeal disease (pCSI)
    - KPS > 70 breast and lung
  - Skull base tumors
    - Benign and malignant
  - Re-irradiation
    - Appropriate functional status
  - Young patients with low-grade gliomas
  - Extensive dural disease
- Can be considered for
  - Leptomeningeal disease (pCSI)
    - KPS > 70 (non-breast, non-lung, case by case)
  - Primary tumors abutting/nearly abutting optic structures and brainstem
    - Due to re-irradiation considerations
  - High-grade gliomas
  - Low-grade gliomas

Pending NRG BN005
- Meningiomas
- Ependymomas
- Posterior fossa tumors
- Calvarial metastases
  Parenchymal sparing in young, good prognostic patients
- Not typically considered for
  - Brain metastases
  - Vestibular schwannomas

References

1. Stupp R, et al. Radiotherapy plus concomitant and adjuvant temozolomide for glioblastoma. NEJM. 2005;352(10):987–96.
2. Kruser T, et al. NRG brain tumor specialists consensus guidelines for glioblastoma contouring. J Neuro Onc. 2019;143:157–66.
3. Roa W, Brasher PM, Bauman G, et al. Abbreviated course of radiation therapy in older patients with glioblastoma multiforme: a prospective randomized clinical trial. J Clin Oncol. 2004;22:1583–8.
4. Perlow H, et al. Dose-escalated accelerated hypofractionation for elderly or frail patients with a newly diagnosed glioblastoma. J Neuro-Oncology. 2022;156:399–406.
5. Azoulay M, et al. A Phase I/II trial of 5 fraction stereotactic radiosurgery with 5mm margins with concurrent temozolomide in newly diagnosed glioblastoma: primary outcomes. Neuro-Oncology. 2020;22:1182–9.
6. Tsien CI, Pugh SL, Dicker AP, et al. NRG oncology/RTOG1205: a randomized phase II trial of concurrent bevacizumab and reirradiation versus bevacizumab alone as treatment for recurrent glioblastoma. J Clin Oncol. 2023;41:1285–95.
7. Roa W, Kepka L, Kumar N, et al. International Atomic Energy Agency randomized phase III study of radiation therapy in elderly and/or frail patients with newly diagnosed glioblastoma multiforme. J Clin Oncol. 2015;33:4145–50.
8. Halasz L, et al. Radiation Therapy for IDH-Mutant Grade 2 and Grade 3 Diffuse Glioma: An ASTRO Clinical Practice Guideline. Pract Radiat Onco. 2022;12:370–86.
9. Gaebe L, et al. Stereotactic radiosurgery versus whole brain radiotherapy in patients with intracranial metastatic disease and small-cell lung cancer: a systematic review and meta-analysis. Lancet Oncol. 2022;23(7):931–3.
10. Brown PD, Gondi V, Pugh S, et al. Hippocampal avoidance during whole-brain radiotherapy plus memantine for patients with brain metastases: phase III trial NRG Oncology CC001. J Clin Oncol. 2020;38:1019–29.
11. Gondi V, et al. Preservation of memory with conformal avoidance of the hippocampal neural stem-cell compartment during whole brain radiotherapy for brain metastases (RTOG 0933): a phase II multi-institutional trial. J Clin Oncol. 2014;32(34):3810–6.
12. Brown PD, Pugh S, Laack NN, et al. Memantine for the prevention of cognitive dysfunction in patients receiving whole-brain radiotherapy: a randomized, double-blind, placebo-controlled trial. Neuro-Oncology. 2013;15:1429–37.
13. Hughes RT, Masters AH, McTyre ER, et al. Initial SRS for patients with 5-15 brain metastases: results of a multi-institutional experience. Int J Radiat Oncol Biol Phys. 2019;104:1091–8.
14. Minniti G, Scaringi C, Paolini S, et al. Single-fraction versus multifraction (3 x 9 Gy) stereotactic radiosurgery for large (>2 cm) brain metastases: a comparative analysis of local control and risk of radiation-induced brain necrosis. Int J Radiat Oncol Biol Phys. 2016;95:1142–8.

15. Soliman H, Ruschin M, Angelov L, et al. Consensus Contouring Guidelines for postoperative completely resected cavity stereotactic radiosurgery for brain metastases. Int J Radiat Oncol Biol Phys. 2018;100:436–42.
16. Yang JT, et al. Randomized Phase II trial of proton craniospinal irradiation versus photon involved-field radiotherapy for patients with solid tumor leptomeningeal metastasis. Clin Oncol. 2022;40(33):3858–67.

Spine SBRT

2

Boris Mueller, Lei Zhang, Divya Yerramilli, and Josh Yamada

Introduction

The development of highly conformal treatment planning in conjunction with near-real-time 3D pre-treatment imaging has allowed high doses of radiation therapy to be given to almost any anatomic site in five or fewer fractions. This approach, referred to as stereotactic body radiation therapy (SBRT) or stereotactic body ablative radiotherapy (SABR), has enabled exciting developments in managing spine tumors, where excellent tumor control can be achieved while limiting toxicity to normal tissue. For solid tumors of the spine, particularly those histologies that have been resistant to conventionally fractionated radiation, local control is often complicated by the presence of nearby critical normal tissues, such as the spinal cord, cauda equina, esophagus, and brachial and lumbosacral plexuses. These critical structures often have a tolerance to radiation doses that are significantly lower than the doses needed to provide local tumor cure. Thus, SBRT has revolutionized the management of spine tumors, with prospective randomized trials reporting durable tumor control of over 90% with minimal severe toxicity [1]. SBRT has also been shown to be highly effective in controlling disease that has been previously irradiated with very acceptable rates of complications. As emerging data supports ablative radiation therapy for oligometastatic disease, spine radiosurgery has also been instrumental in optimizing oncologic outcomes for appropriate patients.

B. Mueller (✉) · L. Zhang · D. Yerramilli · J. Yamada
Department of Radiation Oncology, Memorial Sloan Kettering Cancer Center, New York, NY, USA
e-mail: muellerb@mskcc.org; zhangl7@mskcc.org; yerramid@mskcc.org; yamadaj@mskcc.org

J. J. Cuaron, L. Z. Braunstein (eds.), *Radiation Oncology Clinical Fundamentals*,
https://doi.org/10.1007/978-3-031-77559-8_2

History and Work-Up

For patients with spinal tumors, applying the neurologic, oncologic, mechanical, and systemic (NOMS) framework can be helpful in determining treatment paradigms and is best done in an integrated multidisciplinary approach involving neurosurgery, radiology, radiation oncology, interventional pain management, and physical medicine and rehabilitation [2].

In brief, there are four aspects of the NOMS framework (Fig. 2.1):

1. **Neurologic**
   - Spine tumors frequently have an impact on a patient's neurologic function.
   - It is essential to assess both the patient's degree of symptoms and the radiographic appearance of the extent of epidural disease using the Bilsky grading system (Fig. 2.2).
   - Symptomatic rapidly progressive myelopathy (Bilsky Grade 3 epidural disease) should almost always undergo urgent decompressive surgery.
   - In cases with less severe epidural cord compression without symptoms of myelopathy, oncologic factors can also be considered in determining the appropriate treatment choice.
   - In cases without an established cancer diagnosis, surgery may be preferred to help obtain tissue for pathologic diagnosis. Tissue diagnosis will also help determine tumor radiosensitivity.

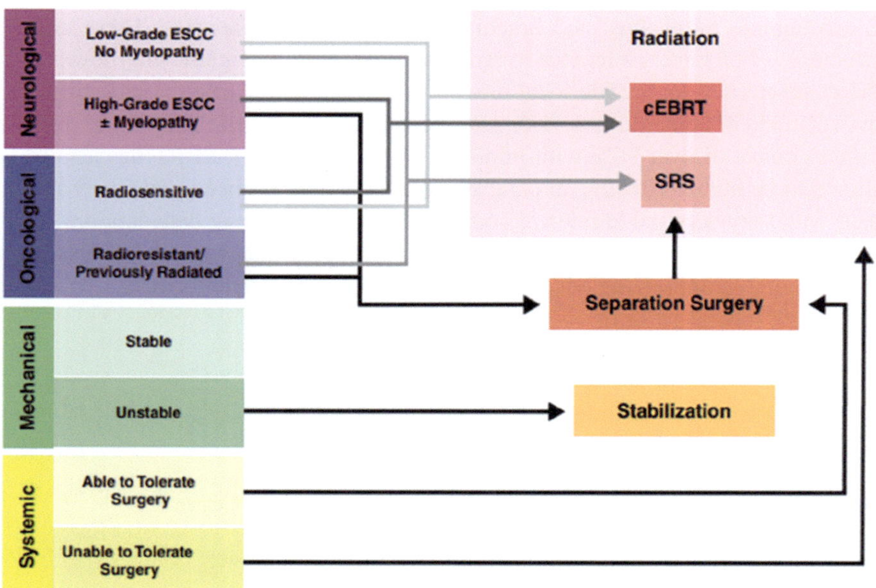

Fig. 2.1 NOMS framework [2]

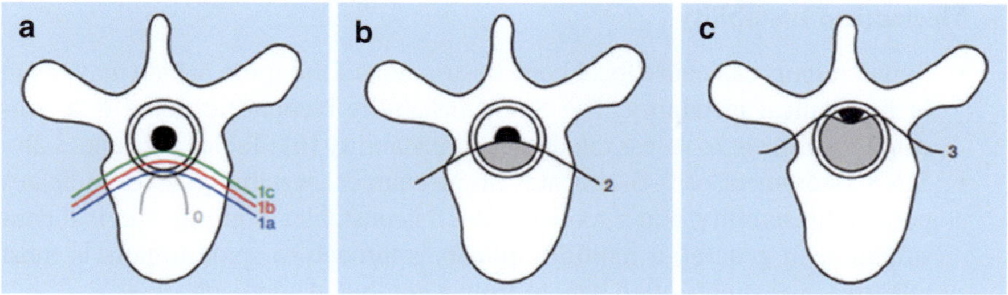

Fig. 2.2 Bilsky grading system [Ref: Bilsky et al., Journal Neurosurgery Spine, 2010]

Table 2.1 Radiation sensitivity by tumor histology

Sensitive	Resistant
Lymphoma	Melanoma
Seminoma	Renal
Myeloma	Non-small cell lung cancer
Breast	Gastrointestinal
Prostate	Gynecologic(not endometrial, not ovarian)
Endometrial	Thyroid
Ovarian	Head & Neck
Thymoma	Urothelial/Bladder
Carcinoid	Sarcoma (not Ewing, not myxoid liposarcoma)
	Any subtype failing radiation

2. **Oncologic**

- The degree of epidural disease is the most important factor in determining the amount of radiation that can be given to a spinal tumor while respecting safe dosimetric constraints to the spinal cord or cauda equina. Typically, mechanically stable patients without myelopathy with radiographic Bilsky Grade 0–2 are considered for definitive radiation therapy without surgery.
- The presumed radiosensitivity is also an important factor in decision-making. Radioresistant tumors such as renal cell carcinoma, non-small cell lung cancer, melanoma, gastrointestinal histologies, and sarcomas are not as likely to durably respond to conventionally fractionated palliative radiotherapy (800 cGy × 1, 400 cGy × 5, 300 cGy × 10), and have superior long-term outcomes when using SBRT techniques (900–1000 cGy × 3, 800 cGy × 5, 1800–2400 cGy × 1 [3]. This is supported by the National Comprehensive Cancer Network (NCCN) guidelines in the management of metastatic spine tumors [4]. Radiosensitive tumors, including breast cancer, prostate cancer, seminomas, and lymphomas, may be well treated with conventionally fractionated radiation therapy (see Table 2.1). All tumors that have recurred after prior radiation therapy are considered radioresistant.
- Separation surgery [5] should be considered when there is extensive radioresistant epidural disease, particularly Bilsky Grade 2 or higher.

3. **Mechanical Instability**

   - Spinal tumors can cause local bony destruction of the spine, which may result in mechanical instability. The Spine Instability Neoplastic Score is a validated instrument to assess the degree of instability [6] (Tables 2.2a and 2.2b).
   - SINS assessment of 0–6 indicates no mechanical instability, 7–12 indicates potential instability, and a score of 13–18 is unstable, requiring surgical consultation. In general, a multidisciplinary approach to spine tumors is most effective, as patients often benefit from a combined approach.
   - Mechanical radiculopathy may also be an indication for surgical intervention. While radiculopathy secondary to nerve impingement from a tumor may respond to radiotherapy, a retropulsed bone fragment or impingement secondary to a pedicle fracture will likely require surgery to palliate.

4. **Systemic**

   - A patient's prognosis is essential to medical decision-making regarding surgical intervention and choice of radiotherapy technique.
   - Prognosis can be informed by performance status, comorbidities informing medical fitness, the burden of systemic disease, the velocity of disease progression, and the availability of further systemic options.

Table 2.2a Spinal Instability Neoplastic Score (SINS) system [7]

Component	Score
Location	
Junctional (O-C2; C7-T2; T11-L1; L5-S1)	3
Mobile spine (C3–6; L2–4)	2
Semirigid (T3–10)	1
Rigid (S2-S5)	0
Mechanical pain	
Yes	3
No	2
Pain-free lesion	1
Bone lesion	
Lytic	2
Mixed (lytic/blastic)	1
Blastic	0
Radiographic spinal alignment	
Subluxation/translation present	4
Deformity (kyphosis/scoliosis)	2
Normal	0
Vertebral body collapse	
>50% collapse	3
<50% collapse	2
No collapse with >50% body involved	1
None of the above	0
Posterolateral involvement	
Bilateral	3
Unilateral	1
None of the above	0

Table 2.2b Total Spinal Instability Neoplastic Score: Determination of stability [7]

Score (Total = 0–18)		
0–6	7–12	13–18
Stable spine	Potentially unstable	Unstable spine

- Patients who are medically ineligible for surgery may rely on radiation therapy as their sole option for both palliative and local control endpoints, and the technique should be chosen appropriately.
- Patients with limited expected survival (<3 months) may be adequately palliated with a short course of conventional radiation (800 cGy × 1).
- Given that patients with metastatic disease are living longer with improved systemic therapies and better stratification, those with a favorable expected survival may benefit from SBRT, with the goal of tumor ablation.

Imaging

During a consultation, an MRI of the entire spine with and without contrast should be obtained. MRI, with a diagnostic accuracy of 98.7%, is superior to CT and PET imaging for identifying spine metastases [8]. Comprehensive evaluation with a total spine MRI is recommended in order to assess for any other synchronous spinal tumors.

If a patient cannot tolerate an MRI due to pain or other factors, sedation can be used. If a patient has implants or pacemakers incompatible with an MRI, a combination of CT of the total spine, PET/CT, or myelogram can be helpful in visualizing mechanical stability, active disease, and degree of epidural disease, respectively.

Simulation

For the majority of patients, CT simulation is done using technique-specific immobilization. Rigid stereotactic immobilization is necessary for SBRT, while simpler immobilization techniques may be appropriate for conventional spinal radiation therapy (Fig. 2.3). For certain paraspinal tumors, particularly with extraosseous extension, such as cervical spine tumors, which may encase vasculature, IV contrast may be helpful in tumor delineation. For certain lumbar spine or sacrum cases where the tumor is close to the small bowel, small bowel contrast can also be helpful. The scan is done using 1–2 mm slices.

Visualization of the spinal cord is equally important in spine tumor management as delineation of the tumor. As such, there are two general approaches to cord delineation. A CT myelogram is a procedure in which iodinated contrast is instilled into the thecal sac, thereby allowing clear visualization of the spinal cord, thecal sac, and epidural disease. However, not all patients are appropriate for a CT myelogram.

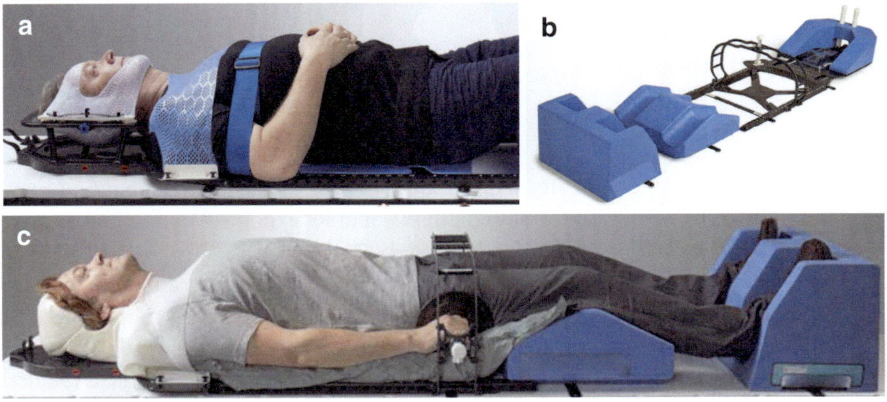

Fig. 2.3 Rigid immobilization for spine SBRT [images provided by CDR systems]. (**a**) 5-point aquaplast mask for cervical spine cases. (**b**) Spine frame for spine SBRT. (**c**) Cradle and frame for thoracic and lumbar cases

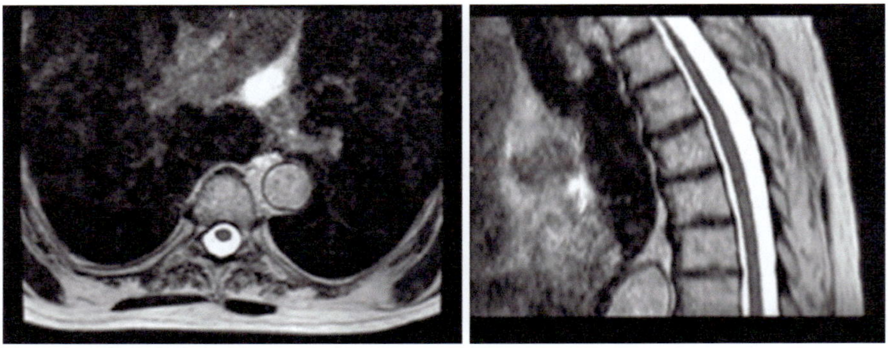

Fig. 2.4 Example of focal spine MRI (3D Axial T2-weighted cube series; MSK Radiology)

Patients require complete blood count, comprehensive metabolic panel, prothrombin time, and international normalized ratio (PT/INR) within 30 days of the myelogram, and anticoagulation must be held before the myelogram procedure. If a patient has increased intracranial pressure with a risk of herniation, hypercapnia, anaphylactic reactions to iodinated CT contrast, or active infection, a myelogram is contraindicated.

In cases where a patient cannot undergo a myelogram, a 3D high-resolution spine MRI is a good option for visualization of the spinal cord, cauda equina nerve roots, thecal sac, and epidural disease. An MRI study that is specifically tailored for spine SBRT treatment planning (images are acquired orthogonally to the imaging couch to match simulation acquisition) and scans one vertebral body above and below the target area (thin slice 3D axial pre- and post-T1, 3D axial T2—Fig. 2.4). Thus, this is best applied to areas of the rigid spine or limited levels of disease. Given the MRI is fused to a CT simulation, a PRV (Planning Risk Volume) expansion of 1–2 mm on the spinal cord should be used for treatment planning.

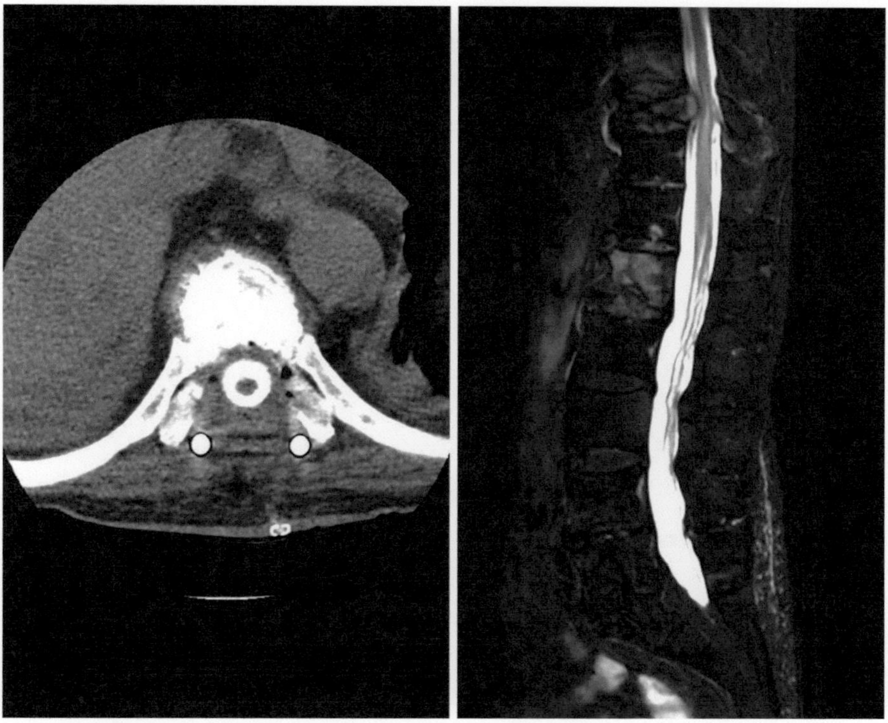

Fig. 2.5 Postoperative CT myelogram (MSK Radiology)

For patients undergoing separation surgery who require postoperative SBRT, simulation can be done on the same admission before patient discharge, given that the bony anatomy and the areas at risk are unlikely to change (Fig. 2.5). Metal artifact reduction can be helpful for simulation imaging.

Contouring

Definitive Cases

The following target volumes should be drawn in accordance with the ISRC Consortium Anatomic Classification System for Consensus Target Volumes for Spine SRS [9]. The GTV should be drawn to include the gross disease in the vertebra, any epidural extension, and paraspinal extension on both the CT and MRI images. For the CTV, the vertebral body is divided into six anatomic compartments (Fig. 2.6). The CTV should include any involved compartments and one adjacent normal bony space to account for subclinical spread. Recent guidelines have also delineated similar compartments for the sacrum (Fig. 2.7) [10]. The PTV should be a 2–3 mm uniform expansion, excluding the thecal sac, and per physician

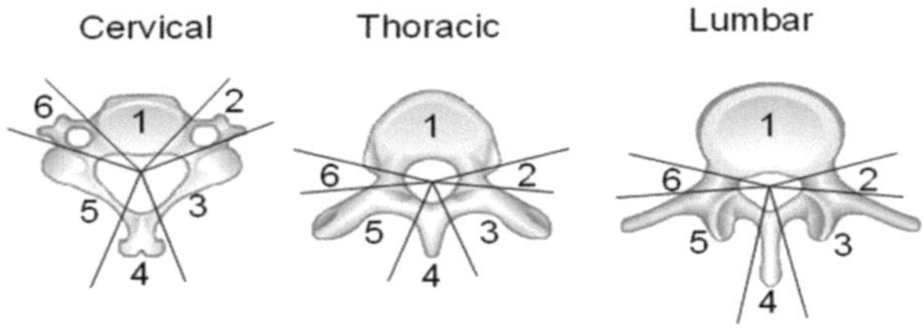

Fig. 2.6 Anatomic divisions of the vertebral body [8]

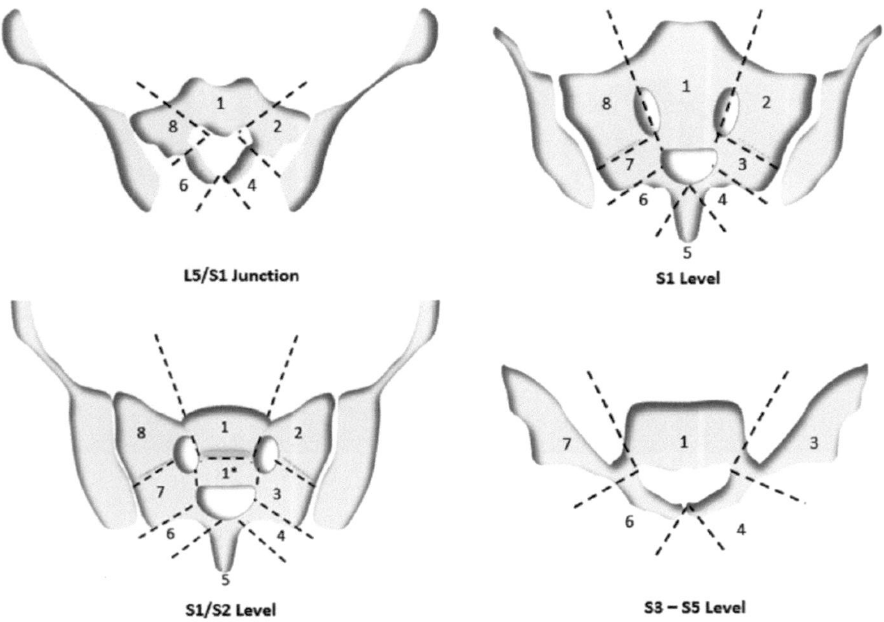

Fig. 2.7 Anatomic divisions of the sacrum [9]

discretion, can exclude the overlapping esophagus. In cases of MR fusion for cord and cauda delineation, a 1 mm expansion should be used to create a spinal cord and cauda PRV. This will account for uncertainties related to MRI/CT fusion and image distortion on MRI.

Whenever possible, target contours should be reviewed in a multidisciplinary fashion.

Postoperative Cases

For postoperative cases, the pre-surgical MRI should be used to identify all bony and paraspinal components involved. The GTV should include all gross disease on the postoperative CT and MRI, including residual epidural disease and paraspinal components of the tumor. CTV should include the GTV, the entire anatomic compartments corresponding to the areas suspicious for tumor noted on the preoperative MRI, and any additional postoperative areas suspicious for tumor. The surgical hardware or the incision sites do not need to be included in the postoperative CTVs. If there is a paraspinal or epidural tumor, additional anatomic expansions up to 5 mm can be considered into paraspinal tissues and craniocaudally along the epidural space. The PTV is created from a 2–3 mm uniform expansion from the CTV, excluding the thecal sac and, in certain cases, excluding sensitive mucosal structures such as the esophagus and small bowel.

Dose/Fractionation

For durable local control in patients with good performance status, such as patients with oligometastatic disease, and for radioresistant histologies, ASTRO guidelines support the use of spine SBRT [11]. Studies comparing SBRT to conventional fractionation have shown variable results, with two negative studies and one positive study, but these studies have heterogeneous populations, with RTOG/NRG 0613, in particular, representing patients with a poor prognosis [12]. A randomized trial of oligometastatic patients has shown local control rates greater than 90% with the use of 24 Gy × 1 [1]. For multilevel vertebral body involvement, particularly if there is an insufficient distance from the spinal cord or mucosal structures, hypofractionated regimens may be appropriate, with 8–10 Gy × 3 or 6–8 Gy × 5 commonly used.

For conventional palliative endpoints, such as pain control and symptomatic relief of cord compression in a palliative setting, multiple randomized trials have supported the use of 8 Gy × 1 compared to longer multi-fraction endpoints such as 3 Gy × 10 fractions, with the only differences noted as higher rates of retreatment in the single-fraction 8 Gy × 1 arm [13]. ASTRO's Choosing Wisely Campaign [14] has advocated for 8 Gy × 1 as a preferred treatment option for poor prognosis patients. With patient convenience in mind, MSKCC, for conventional radiation has generally favored the use of 5 fractions or fewer, with the idea that if dose-escalation is appropriate, SBRT is an appropriate choice of treatment.

In cases of reirradiation after prior conventional radiotherapy, hypofractionated treatment using 9–10 Gy in 3 fractions is typically considered. For patients requiring reirradiation after SBRT recurrence, 8 Gy × 5 with SBRT planning is an effective and safe strategy with sufficient distance from the cord or cauda equina [15]. A time interval of at least 3 months between courses of radiation is preferred.

Planning and Treatment Delivery

Once volumes are completed, planning objectives predominantly include target coverage and respecting OAR (organs at risk) coverage, the most critical of which are mucosal structures and the spinal cord and cauda equina. Ideally, the minimum dose to the CTV is >15 Gy for single-fraction treatments, >21 Gy for 3-fraction therapy, and >25 Gy for 5-fraction therapy.

Paramount to treatment planning is sparing the spinal cord, and for 1-, 3-, and 5-fractions, respectively, the maximum dose to 0.35 cc of the spinal cord should be 10 Gy, 18 Gy, and 23 Gy. In certain cases, particularly where the patient is not a surgical candidate and tumor abuts the spinal cord, these guidelines cannot always be met. Thus, there are spinal cord transection constraints, in which the dose should not traverse the cord contour on any axial slice. Tables 2.3 and 2.4 provide a summary of planning target and normal tissue constraints for both de novo and re-irradiation spine SBRT cases.

Table 2.3 Dosimetric guidelines for treatment planning—for de Novo spine cases

		1-Fraction	3-Fractions	5-Fractions
	Prescription dose	24 Gy × 1	9–10 Gy × 3	8 Gy × 5
Target coverage	PTV coverage	PTV $V_{100\%} \geq 90\%$ and PTV $V_{95\%} \geq 95\%$ (ideal) PTV $V_{100\%} \geq 80\%$ and PTV $V_{95\%} \geq 90\%$ (acceptable)		
	Minimum CTV coverage[a] (ideal)	$DC_{0.035cc} \geq 15$ Gy	$DC_{0.035cc} \geq 21$ Gy	$DC_{0.035cc} \geq 25$ Gy
	Minimum GTV coverage[a] (acceptable)	$DC_{0.035cc} \geq 15$ Gy	$DC_{0.035cc} \geq 21$ Gy	$DC_{0.035cc} \geq 25$ Gy
Neurologic constraints	Spinal cord (PRV if MRI fusion)	$D_{max} < 14$ Gy or 12 Gy[b] $D_{0.35cc} < 10$ Gy	$D_{max} < 26$ Gy or 24 Gy[b] $D_{0.35cc} < 18$ Gy	$D_{max} < 30$ Gy $D_{0.35cc} < 23$ Gy
	Spinal cord transection constraint	10 Gy	18 Gy	23 Gy
	Cauda Equina	$D_{max} < 18$ Gy $D_{5cc} < 14$ Gy	$D_{max} < 26$ Gy $D_{5cc} < 22$ Gy	$D_{max} < 35$ Gy $D_{5cc} < 30$ Gy
	Brachial plexus	$D_{max} < 24$ Gy[c]	$D_{max} < 27$ Gy[c]	$D_{max} < 35$ Gy[c]
	Lumbosacral plexus	No hot spot	$D_{max} < 27$ Gy[c]	$D_{max} < 35$ Gy[c]
Mucosal constraints	Esophagus[d]	Level I: $V_{14Gy} < 2.5$ cc Level II: $V_{18\,Gy} < 2.5$ cc	Level I: $D_{0.035cc} < 27.6$ Gy $D_{5cc} < 16.8$ Gy Level II: $D_{0.035cc} < 30$ Gy $D_{5cc} < 22$ Gy	Level I: $D_{0.035cc} < 32.2$ Gy $D_{5cc} < 19$ Gy Level II: $D_{0.035cc} < 50$ Gy $D_{5cc} < 27.5$ Gy
	Stomach	$D_{max} < 15$ Gy $D_{5cc} < 12$ Gy	$D_{max} < 27$ Gy or 30 Gy[e] $D_{5cc} < 21$ Gy	$D_{max} < 30$ Gy or 33 Gy[e] $D_{5cc} < 25$ Gy
	Small bowel	$D_{max} < 16$ Gy $D_{5cc} < 12$ Gy	$D_{max} < 27$ Gy or 30 Gy[e] $D_{5cc} < 21$ Gy	$D_{max} < 30$ Gy or 33 Gy[e] $D_{5cc} < 25$ Gy $V_{20Gy} < 100$ cc

[a]Use the near-minimum absorbed dose metric $DC_{0.035cc}$, i.e., max dose to the coolest 0.035 cc
[b]Use the lower value if PTV is circumferential
[c]Applies only to portions 3 mm away from the PTV. The portion inside the PTV is limited to 110% of Rx
[d]Attempt level I constraints first. Use level II constraints if level I compromises coverage
[e]User the higher value if overlapping with PTV

Table 2.4 Dosimetric guidelines for treatment planning—for re-irradiation (with one course of prior radiation only, treated at least three months before)

		1-Fraction	3-Fractions	5-Fractions
Neurologic constraints	Spinal cord (PRV if MRI fusion)[a]	D_{max} < 12 Gy Or 10.2 Gy[b] $D_{0.35cc}$ < 9 Gy	D_{max} < 14.5 Gy Or 13.9 Gy[b] $D_{0.35cc}$ < 10 Gy	D_{max} < 18 Gy Or 17 Gy[b] $D_{0.35cc}$ < 14 Gy
	Cauda Equina[a]	D_{max} < 14 Gy D_{5cc} < 11 Gy	D_{max} < 15 Gy D_{5cc} < 13 Gy	D_{max} < 20 Gy D_{5cc} < 17 Gy
	Brachial plexus	No hot spot	D_{max} < 17.7 Gy[c]	D_{max} < 22 Gy[c]
	Lumbosacral plexus	No hot spot	D_{max} < 17.7 Gy[c]	D_{max} < 22 Gy[c]
Mucosal constraints	Esophagus[d]	No hot spot	$D_{0.035cc}$ < 20.4 Gy Cumulative $D_{0.035cc}$ < 100 Gy in 2 Gy equivalents ($\alpha/\beta = 3$)	$D_{0.035cc}$ < 25 Gy Cumulative $D_{0.035cc}$ < 100 Gy in 2 Gy equivalents ($\alpha/\beta = 3$)
	Stomach/small Bowel[d]	No hot spot	Cumulative D_{5cc} < 85 Gy in 2 Gy equivalents ($\alpha/\beta = 3$) Cumulative D_{max} < 65 Gy in 2 Gy equivalents ($\alpha/\beta = 3$)	Cumulative D_{5cc} < 85 Gy in 2 Gy equivalents ($\alpha/\beta = 3$) Cumulative D_{max} < 65 Gy in 2 Gy equivalents ($\alpha/\beta = 3$)

[a]To use the spinal cord or cauda equina re-irradiation constraints, the Rx of prior conventional treatment should not exceed 30 Gy in 10 fractions or 50 Gy in 25 fractions; or the spinal cord D_{max} from prior SBRT should not exceed 14 Gy in 1 fraction, 21 Gy in 3 fractions, or 26 Gy in 5 fractions; the cauda D_{max} from prior SBRT should not exceed 18 Gy in 1 fraction, 26 Gy in 3 fractions, or 30 Gy in 5 fractions

[b]Use the lower value if PTV is circumferential

[c]Apply only to portions 3 mm away from the PTV. The portion inside the PTV is limited to 110% of Rx

[d]The cumulative constraints are total equivalent doses in 2 Gy fractions over prior and current courses of radiation

For mucosal structures such as the esophagus and small bowel include max point dose constraints and maximum dose to a volume of 5 cc (see Tables 2.3 and 2.4).

Treatment planning and delivery typically utilize intensity-modulated radiotherapy (IMRT) with coplanar beams or arc therapy (VMAT) techniques to achieve the desired target coverage with highly conformal dose distribution around the PTV and sharp dose falloff to the spinal cord and other OARs. For each treatment, the patient is positioned under image guidance with kV and cone-beam CT to align the targeted vertebral level and the hardware (if present) according to the planned CT. Intrafractional monitoring with radiographic imaging using an onboard imager or other in-room X-ray imaging system could help ensure patient alignment throughout the treatment and minimize motion-induced dose uncertainties to target and critical organs nearby.

On-Treatment Management and Follow-Up Care

During treatment, patients can expect to be immobilized for approximately 45 minutes to over an hour, depending on the number of sites treated, given the need for alignment, pre-treatment imaging with daily kV X-rays and cone-beam CT requiring physician approval, and delivery of multiple beam angles of therapy with on-board imaging. Radiation-sensitizing agents should typically be held during radiotherapy, although the data regarding concurrent use of immunotherapy, chemotherapy, and targeted agents during palliative radiation or SBRT is not robust. Patients may acutely experience fatigue, pain flare, and discomfort during the therapy, so optimal pain management is crucial for precise immobilization and set-up. For pain flares, anti-inflammatory agents, particularly steroid medications, can be helpful, and patients with symptomatic cord compression are often reflexively started on steroids regardless. With prolonged steroid use, PCP and GI prophylaxis should also be initiated.

During treatment, or afterward, pharyngitis or mucositis is common, given the radiation sensitivity of the esophagus, and can be managed with sucralfate or viscous lidocaine and will gradually resolve with supportive medications. For thoracic or high lumbar lesions, nausea is also possible, for which pre-medication with anti-emetics can be helpful. Less likely are diarrhea or short-term effects on bowel or bladder function for lumbosacral lesions.

Late complications of radiation therapy are rare but serious and include esophageal perforation and/or fistula, pneumonitis, bowel perforation, myelopathy, and damage to the nerve roots. Respecting the OAR tolerances and adequate contouring and planning are designed in such a way to minimize the likelihood of these events. However, the use of concurrent therapies, particularly VEG-F inhibitors, can make the risks of these events unknown and encourage caution in concurrent treatment.

Notably, vertebral compression fractures happen with some frequency, given that the vertebra itself is the target volume. In the literature, symptomatic has been variably reported to be less than 10%. Vertebral compression fractures can occur in the setting of an active tumor or after therapy, but it is an expert consensus opinion that it is easier to manage when the tumor is completely treated, as kyphoplasty can be done to relieve symptoms with a good and instantaneous effect.

Regarding follow-up care, patients may experience pain relief and/or toxicity in the weeks after radiation therapy, so it is important to carefully counsel patients and offer anticipatory guidance regarding these side effects. The NCCN guidelines also support surveillance with repeat spine MRIs every three months, although this must be adjusted according to patient prognosis. Surveillance is particularly important as patients with metastatic spinal disease commonly require additional treatment courses at other levels of the spine. In the long term, it can be essential for patients to work with physical and occupational therapy, particularly if they present with symptoms concerning myelopathy.

References

1. Zelefsky MJ, Yamada Y, Greco C, Lis E, Schöder H, Lobaugh S, Zhang Z, Braunstein S, Bilsky MH, Powell SN, Kolesnick R, Fuks Z. Phase 3 multi-center, prospective, randomized trial comparing single-dose 24 Gy radiation therapy to a 3-fraction SBRT regimen in the treatment of oligometastatic cancer. Int J Radiat Oncol Biol Phys. 2021;110(3):672–9. https://doi.org/10.1016/j.ijrobp.2021.01.004. Epub 2021 Jan 8.
2. Laufer I, Rubin DG, Lis E, Cox BW, Stubblefield MD, Yamada Y, Bilsky MH. The NOMS framework: approach to the treatment of spinal metastatic tumors. Oncologist. 2013;18(6):744–51. https://doi.org/10.1634/theoncologist.2012-0293.
3. Yamada Y, Katsoulakis E, Laufer I, Lovelock M, Barzilai O, McLaughlin LA, Zhang Z, Schmitt AM, Higginson DS, Lis E, Zelefsky MJ, Mechalakos J, Bilsky MH. The impact of histology and delivered dose on local control of spinal metastases treated with stereotactic radiosurgery. Neurosurg Focus. 2017;42(1):E6.
4. National Comprehensive Cancer Network, Central Nervous System Cancers, Version 1.2024. https://www.nccn.org/professionals/physician_gls/pdf/cns.pdf, 31 May 2024.
5. Moussazadeh N, Laufer I, Yamada Y, Bilsky MH. Separation surgery for spinal metastases: effect of spinal radiosurgery on surgical treatment goals. Cancer Control. 2014;21(2):168–74. https://doi.org/10.1177/107327481402100210.
6. Fourney DR, Frangou EM, Ryken TC, DiPaola CP, Shaffrey CI, Berven SH, Bilsky MH, Harrop JS, Fehlings MG, Boriani S, Chou D, Schmidt MH, Polly DW, Biagini R, Burch S, Dekutoski MB, Ganju A, Gerszten PC, Gokaslan ZL, et al. Spinal instability neoplastic score: an analysis of reliability and validity from the spine Oncology Study Group. J Clin Oncol. 2011;29(22):3072–7. https://doi.org/10.1200/JCO.2010.34.3897.
7. Fisher CG, DiPaola CP, Ryken TC, et al. A novel classification system for spinal instability in neoplastic disease: an evidence-based approach and expert consensus from the Spine Oncology Study Group. Spine(Phila Pa 1976). 2010;35:E1221–9.
8. Buhmann Kirchhoff S, Becker C, Duerr HR, Reiser M, Baur-Melnyk A. Detection of osseous metastases of the spine: comparison of high resolution multi-detector-CT with MRI. Eur J Radiol. 2009;69(3):567–73. https://doi.org/10.1016/j.ejrad.2007.11.039. Epub 2008 Jan 11.
9. Cox BW, Spratt DE, Lovelock M, Bilsky MH, Lis E, Ryu S, Sheehan J, Gerszten PC, Chang E, Gibbs I, Soltys S, Sahgal A, Deasy J, Flickinger J, Quader M, Mindea S, Yamada Y. International spine radiosurgery consortium consensus guidelines for target volume definition in spinal stereotactic radiosurgery. Int J Radiat Oncol Biol Phys. 2012;83(5):e597–605. https://doi.org/10.1016/j.ijrobp.2012.03.009. Epub 2012 May 19.
10. Dunne EM, Sahgal A, Lo SS, Bergman A, Kosztyla R, Dea N, Chang EL, Chang U-K, Chao ST, Faruqi S, Ghia AJ, Redmond KJ, Soltys SG, Liu MC. International consensus recommendations for target volume delineation specific to sacral metastases and spinal stereotactic body radiation therapy (SBRT). Radiother Oncol. 2020;145:21–9. https://doi.org/10.1016/j.radonc.2019.11.026. Epub 2019 Dec 23.PMID: 31874346.
11. Alcorn S, Cortés ÁA, Bradfield L, Brennan M, Dennis K, Diaz DA, Doung Y-C, Elmore S, Hertan L, Johnstone C, Jones J, Larrier N, Lo SS, Nguyen Q-N, Tseng YD, Yerramilli D, Zaky S, Balboni T. External beam radiation therapy for palliation of symptomatic bone metastases: an ASTRO Clinical Practice Guideline. Pract Radiat Oncol. 2024;14(5):377–97. https://doi.org/10.1016/j.prro.2024.04.018.
12. Ryu S, Deshmukh S, Timmerman RD, Movsas B, Gerszten P, Yin FF, Dicker A, Abraham CD, Zhong J, Shiao SL, Tuli R, Desai A, Mell LK, Iyengar P, Hitchcock YJ, Allen AM, Burton S, Brown D, Sharp HJ, Dunlap NE, Siddiqui MS, Chen TH, Pugh SL, Kachnic LA. Stereotactic radiosurgery vs conventional radiotherapy for localized vertebral metastases of the spine: phase 3 results of NRG oncology/RTOG 0631 randomized clinical trial. JAMA Oncol. 2023;9(6):800–7. https://doi.org/10.1001/jamaoncol.2023.0356. PMID: 37079324; PMCID: PMC10119775.

13. Hartsell WF, Scott CB, Bruner DW, Scarantino CW, Ivker RA, Roach M 3rd, Suh JH, Demas WF, Movsas B, Petersen IA, Konski AA, Cleeland CS, Janjan NA, DeSilvio M. Randomized trial of short- versus long-course radiotherapy for palliation of painful bone metastases. J Natl Cancer Inst. 2005;97(11):798–804. https://doi.org/10.1093/jnci/dji139.
14. Hahn C, Kavanagh B, Bhatnagar A, Jacobson G, Lutz S, Patton C, Potters L, Steinberg M, Wisely C. The American Society for Radiation Oncology's Top 5 list. Pract Radiat Oncol. 2014;4(6):349–55. https://doi.org/10.1016/j.prro.2014.06.003.
15. Moore A, Zhang Z, Fei T, Zhang L, Accomando L, Schmitt AM, Higginson DS, Mueller BA, Zinovoy M, Gelblum DY, Yerramilli D, Xu AJ, Brennan VS, Guttmann DM, Grossman CE, Dover LL, Shaverdian N, Pike LRG, Cuaron JJ, Dreyfuss A, Lis E, Barzilai O, Bilsky MH, Yamada Y. 40 gray in 5 fractions for salvage reirradiation of spine lesions previously treated with stereotactic body radiotherapy. Neurosurgery. 2024;95(2):380–91. https://doi.org/10.1227/neu.0000000000002889. Epub 2024 Mar 8. PMID: 38456696.

Head and Neck Cancers

3

Nancy Lee and Yingzhi Wu

Workup

Workup of head and neck cancers includes a complete head and neck exam, imaging, and biopsy of the primary site or fine needle aspiration (FNA) of the cervical lymph node. Flexible nasopharyngoscopy is performed to evaluate pharynx (nasopharynx, oropharynx, and hypopharynx) and larynx cancers.

Imaging plays an important role in head and neck cancer staging. IV contrast is preferred if there is no contraindication. 18-Fluoro-deoxyglucose (FDG) PET/CT is usually used to help evaluate distant metastases and detect primary sites if the primary site is not obviously shown on cross-sectional imaging. MRI is preferred over CT to evaluate oral tongue invasion from oropharynx cancer, skull base invasion from nasopharynx cancer and sinonasal cancer, and perineural invasion. CT is helpful to evaluate cartilage invasion from larynx cancer and any bony invasion.

Once radiation therapy is recommended, the patient should be referred to a dental oncologist as soon as possible for a comprehensive dental evaluation and treatments for active dental caries or periodontal disease. In addition, the patient should have a baseline swallowing evaluation and receive individualized instructions for swallowing exercise. If the patient has experienced weight loss at diagnosis, a referral to a nutritionist should be made.

N. Lee (✉) · Y. Wu
Department of Radiation Oncology, Memorial Sloan Kettering Cancer Center, New York, NY, USA
e-mail: leen2@MSKCC.ORG; wuy2@mskcc.org

J. J. Cuaron, L. Z. Braunstein (eds.), *Radiation Oncology Clinical Fundamentals*,
https://doi.org/10.1007/978-3-031-77559-8_3

Simulation

An open face, 3- or 5-point mashed mask is used to secure the treatment position. PET/CT/MR simulation with IV contrast is preferred. If only CT simulation (CT SIM) with intravenous contrast (IV contrast) is performed, diagnostic FDG PET/CT and MRI should be used for fusion in target delineation.

If tooth extraction is recommended, it should be completed at least 1 week prior to simulation to allow healing. If tooth extraction is performed after simulation, repeat simulation is needed due to anatomy changes.

Cancer of Unknown Primary

Head and neck cancer of unknown primary accounts for about 5% [1]. The patient presents with enlarged cervical lymph node(s), which is biopsy-proven positive for metastatic carcinoma, without the primary site identified. Workup including high-risk HPV testing, Epstein–Barr virus (EBV) testing, imaging, and an exam under anesthesia (EUA) should be completed in efforts to identify the primary site. FDG PET/CT is useful to reveal the primary site, which may not be appreciated on CT or MRI. Exam under anesthesia (EUA) enables thorough examination of mucosa and biopsy of suspicious mucosal abnormalities. It is recommended that at least ipsilateral tonsillectomy be done in search of the primary tumor site.

The most common histology of head and neck cancer of unknown primary is squamous cell carcinoma [1]. Treatment is either neck dissection or a radiation therapy (RT)-based approach. Postoperative adjuvant therapy is given depending on pathologic findings. HPV-related head and neck cancer of unknown primary is usually treated as oropharynx cancer. EBV-related head and neck cancer of unknown primary is usually treated as nasopharynx cancer.

Oropharyngeal Cancer

Evidenced by the Gillison et al. study, about 25% of head and neck squamous cell carcinomas (HNSCCs) are casually associated with HPV infection, predominantly oropharyngeal squamous cell carcinoma that arises from lingual or palatine tonsils with poor differentiation and basaloid morphology [2]. This subgroup of HNSCCs, mediated by HPV, have markedly different risk factors from HPV-negative HNSCCs. Another study by Gillison et al. showed several measures of sexual behavior and exposure to marijuana were associated with HPV-positive HNSCCs, while tobacco and alcohol use and poor oral hygiene were associated with HPV-negative HNSCCs [3]. Thus, HPV-positive oropharynx cancer and HPV-negative oropharynx cancer are different diseases and now have different staging criteria in the AJCC eighth edition staging. HPV testing, such as p16 IHC and HPV ISH, is recommended in all patients diagnosed with oropharynx cancer.

Early-stage oropharynx cancer can be treated with either surgery or definitive radiation therapy (RT). The ORATOR trial, which studied swallowing-related quality of life (QOL) scores in patients with early-stage oropharynx cancer treated with transoral robotic surgery (TORS) with neck dissection +/− adjuvant therapy versus definitive RT +/− chemotherapy, reported similar overall survival (OS) and progression-free survival (PFS) in both groups [4]. Swallowing-related QOL in the definitive RT group was superior to the TORS group, but the difference was not a clinically meaningful change, and the difference was decreasing over time [5].

Treatment for locally advanced oropharynx cancer is either surgery followed by adjuvant RT +/− chemotherapy based on pathologic findings or definitive chemoRT. If the surgery approach will require adjuvant chemoRT, definitive chemoRT is preferred given increased toxicity from triple modality management. High-dose cisplatin is the preferred chemotherapy agent in the definitive chemoRT approach. When a patient is symptomatic from a tumor, induction chemotherapy can be given to shrink the tumor and relieve the symptoms prior to definitive chemoRT.

Ang et al. analyzed the association between tumor HPV status and survival among patients with Stage III or IV oropharyngeal squamous cell carcinoma treated with chemoRT. It was reported that patients with HPV-positive cancer had better OS and PFS than patients with HPV-negative cancer [6]. Given patients with HPV-positive oropharynx cancer have a better prognosis, multiple studies of different de-escalatory strategies have been conducted to look for a de-intensified treatment regimen that maintains high patient survival but reduces toxicities.

- Can cisplatin be replaced? NO. RTOG 1016 randomized patients with HPV-positive oropharynx cancer to receive either RT plus cetuximab or RT plus cisplatin. The result showed inferior OS and PFS in the RT plus cetuximab group compared with the RT plus cisplatin group [7]. Similarly, in a Phase III study conducted at 32 centers in Ireland, the Netherlands, and the UK, HPV-positive low-risk oropharynx cancer patients were randomized to receive either cisplatin or cetuximab in addition to RT. The difference between two groups in 2-year overall survival and 2-year recurrence was significant, with cisplatin superior to cetuximab [8].
- Can chemotherapy be omitted? NO. NRG Oncology HN002 randomized patients with p16-positive oropharynx cancer to receive either 60 Gy IMRT over 6 weeks with concurrent weekly cisplatin or 60 Gy IMRT over 5 weeks. The chemoRT group met the acceptable criteria for 2-year PFS, while the accelerated RT group did not [9].
- Can the RT dose be reduced? NO. Based on the NRG Oncology announcement that 60Gy RT plus cisplatin was not non-inferior to the standard 70Gy RT plus cisplatin [10]. Therefore, NRG Oncology abandoned using 60Gy to treat HPV+ oropharyngeal carcinoma.
- Can postoperative RT dose be reduced? Perhaps. ECOG 3311 was designed to assess the 2-year PFS of TORS followed by reduced adjuvant RT in patients with intermediated risk (patients without extracapsular extension or positive margin)

by giving HPV+ oropharynx cancer patients risk-adapted adjuvant therapy after TORS. The study reported that TORS followed by 50 Gy IMRT achieved 95% 2-year PFS among patients with intermediate risk [11].

- The major radiation dose de-escalation trial at Memorial Sloan Kettering Cancer Center is delivering 30 Gy RT with 2 cycles of standard chemotherapy to patients with T1-2N1-2c HPV-associated oropharynx squamous cell carcinoma or HPV-associated squamous cell carcinoma with nodal metastases but unknown primary sites if the tumor is hypoxia negative. Riaz et al. reported a 2-year locoregional control rate of 94.4% and overall survival of 94.7% among 19 patients who were enrolled from July 2015 to October 2016 [12]. Updated series showed that indeed, with careful patient selection, 30Gy RT plus cisplatin was able to eradicate the majority of the HPV+ oropharyngeal carcinoma [13].

Oral Cavity

Oral cavity cancers include cancer of buccal mucosa, anterior two thirds of the tongue, floor of mouth, retromolar trigone, alveolar ridge, and hard palate. The area has a rich lymphatic supply. Most nodal involvement is in levels I, II, and III. But the risk for regional nodal involvement varies depending on the site of the primary tumor [1]. For example, nodal involvement is more commonly seen with oral tongue cancer than with hard palate cancer. Compared to AJCC seventh edition staging, AJCC eighth edition is using depth of invasion (DOI) for T staging in addition to the size of the primary tumor. For example, T1 disease per AJCC seventh edition is upgraded to T2 per AJCC eighth edition if DOI is 5–10 mm.

As to treatment, oral cavity cancer is a surgical disease. For early-stage and locally advanced resectable oral cavity cancer, surgery +/− reconstruction is preferred. Postoperative RT +/− chemotherapy is recommended based on disease staging and pathologic adverse features. Adjuvant chemoRT is recommended for adverse features of extracapsular extension (ECE) or positive margin; adjuvant RT is recommended for other risk factors such as perineural invasion (PNI), lymphoavascular invasion (LVI), pT3 primary, pT4 primary, pN2 nodal disease, or pN3 nodal disease.

- Generally, patients with early stage (pT1-2 N0) oral tongue squamous cell carcinoma (OTSCC) have a better prognosis and do not receive adjuvant RT if there are no adverse pathology features. However, Ganly et al. reported higher regional recurrence than expected among patients with low-risk, early-stage OTSCC who didn't receive adjuvant RT; and that the primary tumor thickness of ≥4 mm was the only independent predictor for neck recurrence though tumor thickness is usually not used as a risk factor to recommend adjuvant RT [14]. Most recently, a retrospective cohort study demonstrated improved survival outcomes in the adjuvant RT group with pT1-2 N0 OTSCC, with benefit more notable in patients with moderate-to-poor differentiation, PNI, and/or LVI [15].

- Both EORTC 22931 and RTOG 9501 reported postoperative adjuvant chemoRT had significantly higher locoregional control and disease-free survival than adjuvant RT for locally advanced head and neck cancers [16, 17].
- A comparative analysis of trials EORTC 22931 and RTOG 9501 showed patients with ECE and/or microscopically involved surgical margins had significantly poorer outcomes and that the addition of concurrent chemotherapy to adjuvant RT improved locoregional control and overall survival of locally advanced head and neck cancers with one or both of these adverse features [18].

Nasopharynx Cancer

Nasopharynx cancer is rare worldwide, but it is an endemic disease in some areas, with the highest incidence in Southeast Asia. Among all head and neck cancers, nasopharynx cancer has a higher incidence of distant metastasis. Histologically, nasopharynx cancer has 2 subtypes: keratinizing and non-keratinizing. Epstein–Barr virus (EBV) is etiologically linked to non-keratinizing subtype, which accounts for the majority of cases in endemic areas. EBV testing of the tumor should be performed as part of the workup.

Radiation therapy is the backbone of treatments given the high radiosensitivity of nasopharynx cancer and the location of the nasopharyngeal tumor.

- Stage I (T1N0) nasopharynx cancer is treated with radiation therapy alone.
- Stage II consists of T2N0 and T1-2N1 subgroups. Chinese Society of Clinical Oncology (CSCO) and American Society of Clinical Oncology (ASCO) Guidelines state chemotherapy is not routinely recommended for T2N0 but may be offered if adverse features exist [19]. Concurrent chemoRT may be offered for T1-2N1, especially for T2N1. Chen et al. study reported 5-year OS, PFS, and distant metastasis-free survival significantly improved in patients with Stage II disease who received RT with concurrent weekly cisplatin compared to patients who received RT alone [20] and that the 10-year outcomes of this study showed the survival benefit mainly in patients with T2N1 disease [21].
- Locally advanced (Stage III–IV A) nasopharynx cancer should be treated with RT and chemotherapy. The Phase III randomized intergroup study 0099 was closed early when interim analysis showed 3-year PFS and 3-year OS were higher for the patients who underwent RT with concurrent cisplatin followed by 3 cycles of adjuvant cisplatin and 5-FU than the patients who underwent RT alone [22].

The sequence of the addition of chemotherapy to concurrent chemoRT for patients with locally advanced nasopharynx cancer has been heatedly debated, with multiple studies being conducted and yielding mixed results.

- MAC-NPC meta-analysis updated by Blanchard et al. confirmed that the significant improvement of OS and PFS in patients with locally advanced nasopharynx cancer was associated with the addition of concurrent chemotherapy to radiation therapy but was not able to conclude the benefits of adjuvant chemotherapy following concurrent chemoradiation therapy [23].

- A Phase III multicenter randomized controlled study by Chen et al. showed adjuvant cisplatin and 5-FU did not significantly improve survival following RT with concurrent weekly cisplatin in patients with Stage III or IV (except T3-4N0) nasopharynx cancer [24].
- Zhang et al. compared induction chemotherapy of gemcitabine and cisplatin followed by concurrent chemoRT with concurrent chemoRT alone among patients with locally advanced nasopharynx cancer and reported that the addition of induction chemotherapy to concurrent chemoRT significantly improved recurrence-free survival and overall survival [25].
- Chen et al. studied the benefit of metronomic capecitabine as adjuvant therapy following concurrent chemoRT and reported significantly improved failure-free survival in patients with locally advanced nasopharynx cancer who received adjuvant metronomic capecitabine compared to patients who received definitive chemoRT only [26].
- EBV DNA-directed personalization of locoregionally advanced nasopharyngeal carcinoma is likely going to be the standard of care, although results are not published yet [27]. Awaiting results of NRG HN001 to see if plasma EBV DNA can guide treatment for locoregionally advanced NPC.

Nasal Cavity/Paranasal Cancer

Nasal cavity and paranasal cancer is rare, with maxillary sinus cancer more common [1]. Histologies include squamous cell carcinoma, esthesioneuroblastoma, sinonasal undifferentiated carcinoma, sinonasal neuroendocrine carcinoma, small cell carcinoma, etc.

Early-stage nasal cavity and paranasal cancer can be treated with surgery alone. Locally advanced resectable nasal cavity and panasanal cancer are usually treated with surgery followed by adjuvant RT +/− chemo based on pathologic risk factors. Locally advanced unresectable nasal cavity and panasanal cancer can be treated with definitive chemoRT. Induction chemotherapy may also be recommended to shrink the tumor, followed by surgery or definitive chemoRT, which is decided based on the disease response to induction chemotherapy.

Mimica et al. reviewed patients with Stage III or IV squamous cell carcinoma of the anterior nasal mucosa who refused total rhinectomy and were treated with definitive RT with or without chemotherapy at Memorial Sloan Kettering Cancer Center. The study reported a 2-year rhinectomy-free survival rate of 88% [28].

Larynx Cancer

Subsites of larynx are supraglottis (epiglottis, false cords, arytenoids, aryepiglottic folds, ventricles), glottis (true vocal cords, anterior and posterior commissure), and subglottis. About 2/3 of larynx cases arise from glottic larynx, with about 30% from supraglottic larynx and 5% from subglottic region [1]. Hoarseness usually develops early among glottic cancer patients, so most glottic cancers are at an early stage at diagnosis and rarely have nodal involvement. However, over 50% of supraglottic cases are found to have spread to regional lymph nodes, thus often locally advanced at diagnosis [1].

For early-stage glottic larynx cancer, treatment options are surgery or RT, which have similar effectiveness. When treating early stage glottic larynx cancer with RT, hypofractionation with shorter treatment duration is preferred based on studies that evaluated the influence of fraction size and overall treatment time on local control.

- Yamazaki et al. randomized study showed use of 2.25 Gy fractions with shorter treatment time had better local control rate than 2 Gy fractions without increased acute toxicities for T1N0 glottic cancers [29].
- Le et al. study showed overall treatment time, fraction size, and total dose were significant prognostic factors for T2 glottic cancers. Patients with T2 lesions had the best local control rate when they were treated with fraction size ≥2.25 Gy, had an overall time ≤ 43 days, or had a total dose >65 Gy [30].

The conventional treatment for locally advanced glottic and supraglottic larynx cancers is total laryngectomy, which causes substantial functional morbidity, followed by postoperative RT +/– chemotherapy. Over the past 2 decades, the concept of organ preservation has been being established. In the early 1990s, a VA trial reported that the regimen of induction chemotherapy followed by definitive RT was effective in larynx preservation with similar 2-year survival as surgery and radiation [31]. The RTOG 91–11 trial, the successor to the VA trial, was designed to find out a better non-surgical regimen by comparing induction chemotherapy followed by RT versus concurrent chemoRT versus RT alone. Concurrent chemoRT was confirmed to be superior in larynx preservation and local control [32]. Of note, the RTOG 91–11 trial excluded high-volume T4 primaries. Eita et al. reviewed nonoperative management of T4 laryngeal and hypolaryngeal cancer at Memorial Sloan Kettering Cancer Center and reported better than previously noted outcomes after non-surgical treatments [33].

When patients with locally advanced glottic and supraglottic larynx cancer have persistent or locally recurrent disease following organ preservation therapy, salvage total laryngectomy is usually performed, which was found to have acceptable morbidity, with survival not influenced by prior organ preservation treatments [34].

Hypopharynx Cancer

Subsites of hypopharynx are pyriform sinus, posterior pharyngeal wall, and post cricoid area. The hypopharynx cancers are rare, and the prognosis is poor.

Usually, the tumors are large at diagnosis. The treatments of locally advanced hypopharynx cancer are either surgery followed by RT +/− chemotherapy or an organ preservation approach (similar to larynx cancer). EORTC trial 24,891 compared surgical approach with definitive RT after complete response to induction chemotherapy and reported that induction chemotherapy followed by RT provided equivalent PFS as the surgical approach and allowed organ preservation in over 50% of survivors [35].

General Contouring and PTV Expansion Recommendations

For the primary site, GTV70 is the volume of all known gross disease, which is decided based on imaging and a physical exam (including flexible nasopharyngoscopy if indicated). PTV70 is usually expanded from GTV70 by 5 mm.

For a lymph node, GTV70 is the volume of all gross positive lymph nodes defined as >1 cm in size, with necrotic appearance, or FDG PET avid. PTV70 is usually expanded from GTV70 by 3 mm.

Clinical target volume (CTV), regions at risk for microscopic disease, is decided based on the potential spread routes of primary sites and lymph nodes. Each subsite of head and neck cancers has a different potential spread route; please see Target Volume Delineation for Conformal and Intensity-Modulated Radiation Therapy (Lee, Riaz, Lu Editors) for CTV delineation recommendations of each disease site. PTV70 should be included in CTV. PTV is expanded from CTV by 3–5 mm. Generally, at the primary site, the distance from GTV70 to PTV should be 1.3 cm. The subclinical CTV dose varies. At our center, 30Gy for HPV+ and 40Gy for HPV- is used. Some other centers can treat the subclinical dose to as high as 63Gy. The toxicity is very high from these series versus our lower subclinical dose.

Dosing Schemes

The radiotherapy dose for head and neck cancers varies depending on disease subsite, definitive setting versus postoperative setting, whether concurrent chemo is given, risk of potential spread to the region, HPV status in oropharynx cancer cases, etc.

In the postoperative setting, the standard radiotherapy dose is 60 Gy if there is no ECE or positive margin. 50 Gy can be considered for HPV+ oropharynx cancers with intermediate pathologic risk factors given ECOG 3311 as discussed previously. If ECE and/or positive margin exists, concurrent chemotherapy is needed, with the node with ECE and/or positive margin area boosted to 66 Gy. For HPV-positive oropharynx cancer cases with ECE and/or positive margin, 60 Gy radiotherapy is delivered with concurrent chemotherapy.

In the definitive RT alone setting, the dose for T1N0 larynx cancer is 63Gy in 28 fractions and 65.25 Gy in 29 fractions for T2N0 larynx cancer. The dose for T1-2N0 oropharynx cancer and nasopharynx cancer is 69.96 Gy in 33 fractions.

In the definitive chemoRT setting, the standard dose for elective treatment regions is 50–60 Gy, while the gross disease receives 70 Gy. Given RT-related late toxicity, several studies have been conducted to decrease the dose to the elective volume.

- Deschuymer et al. reported no statistically significant difference in overall survival, local recurrence, or distant metastases between patients who received 40 Gy to elective nodal volume and who received 50 Gy to elective nodal volume during chemoRT [36]. The group of 40 Gy to elective nodal volume had better outcomes regarding global health status, physical functioning, emotional functioning, speech problems, and trouble with social eating, though there was no clinically relevant improvement in QOL [37].
- Since 2017, we have been treating elective volume to 30 Gy for patients with HPV-associated oropharynx cancer undergoing chemoRT at Memorial Sloan Kettering Cancer Center. 2-year follow-up showed favorable disease control and toxicity profile [38].

On Treatment Management

Head and neck RT-induced acute toxicities are substantial, despite advances and innovations in the planning and delivery technologies. Among them, oral mucositis is most debilitating, contributing to pain, dysphagia, weight loss, and possible fungal infection. Dermatitis and increased secretions are another two common acute toxicities. The sequelae of these acute toxicities may lead to hospitalization, treatment interruption, or even treatment discontinuation. Patients should be assessed for acute toxicities at least once a week and when there are any acute changes. It is important to provide patients with optimal symptom management.

- It is suggested that the oral care protocols be performed to prevent oral mucositis. The protocol includes brushing teeth with a soft toothbrush, flossing, and at least 1 minute of non-medicated mouth rinses (saline or sodium bicarbonate rinses) in all age groups through treatments till oral mucositis heals [39].
- Topical anesthetics (such as viscous lidocaine or Magic Mouthwash) are prescribed at the onset of oral mucositis when erythema is noted and the patient reports sensitivity to spicy or acidic food. Gabapentin, short-acting opioids, and long-acting opioids are prescribed as mucositis evolves and pain increases. Temperature should be taken prior to taking Acetaminophen if the patient is undergoing chemotherapy. Diet modification may be recommended.

- Oral candidiasis is the most common fungal infection of the oral cavity. Nystatin is prescribed for mild oral candidiasis, and fluconazole is prescribed for moderate to severe oral candidiasis [40].
- Patient's swallowing function is closely monitored by speech-language pathologist through RT. Patients are encouraged to continue to eat and drink by mouth as well as do swallowing exercise. PEG tube is not prophylactically placed.
- Patient's weight loss and nutritional status should be evaluated every week during RT. The patient is provided with individualized dietary counseling by nutritionists. Oral nutritional supplements are usually recommended to help meet required calorie intake. Feeding tube is considered if patient fails to meet goal of calorie intake.
- The patient is advised to apply moisturizer twice a day to the RT field for skin care. Steroid topical is prescribed to reduce discomfort (such as burning and itching sensation) and erythema from dermatitis. Silvadene is initiated when moist desquamation develops.
- Mucinex or glycopyrrolate is used for symptom relief from increased secretions. A humidifier is also recommended.

Follow-Up Care

After RT is completed, the patient should continue to be closely monitored for acute toxicities until recovery. At Memorial Sloan Kettering Cancer Center, Advanced Practice Providers follow up patients to manage RT side effects until recovery.

3–4 months after RT, a physical exam (including flexible nasopharyngoscopy if indicated) and imaging (usually FDG PET/CT) are performed to evaluate treatment response.

For cancer surveillance, the patient should be examined every 3–4 months within the first 2 years and every 6 months within 3–5 years. Routine surveillance imaging in clinically asymptomatic patients is not standardized. Annual imaging can be considered to visualize the area inaccessible to clinical exam [1].

RT-related long-term side effects should be monitored and managed, such as xerostomia, dysgeusia, trismus, neck fibrosis, etc.

- Dental cleaning every 3–4 months and high-potent fluoride products are recommended to prevent tooth cavities.
- The patient continues to be followed up by the speech-language pathologist as clinically indicated.
- The patient is instructed to do jaw and neck stretching exercises daily. Referral to physical therapy should be made for trismus or decreased neck range of motion when indicated.
- Referral to lymphedema therapy should be made when lymphedema therapy is identified.

Thyroid function (TSH and fT4) is recommended to be checked every 6–12 months and when the patient reports symptoms suspicious for hypothyroidism if the neck is irradiated.

References

1. NCCN Clinical Practice Guidelines in Oncology Head and Neck Cancers Version 1.2025 https://www.nccn.org/professionals/physician_gls/pdf/head-and-neck.pdf.
2. Gillison ML, Koch WM, Capone RB, et al. Evidence for a causal association between human papillomavirus and a subset of head and neck cancers. J Natl Cancer Inst. 2000;92(9):709–20.
3. Gillison ML, D'Souza G, Westra W, et al. Distinct risk factor profiles for human papillomavirus type 16-positive and human papillomavirus type 16-negative head and neck cancers. J Natl Cancer Inst. 2008;100(6):407–20.
4. Nichols AC, Theurer J, Prisman E, et al. Radiotherapy versus transoral robotic surgery and neck dissection for oropharyngeal squamous cell carcinoma (ORATOR): an open-label, phase 2, randomised trial. Lancet Oncol. 2019 Oct;20(10):1349–59.
5. Nichols AC, Theurer J, Prisman E, et al. Randomized trial of radiotherapy versus transoral robotic surgery for oropharyngeal squamous cell carcinoma: long-term results of the ORATOR trial. J Clin Oncol. 2022;40(8):866–75.
6. Ang KK, Harris J, Wheeler R, et al. Human papillomavirus and survival of patients with oropharyngeal cancer. N Engl J Med. 2010;363(1):24–35.
7. Gillison ML, Trotti AM, Harris J, et al. Radiotherapy plus cetuximab or cisplatin in human papillomavirus-positive oropharyngeal cancer (NRG Oncology RTOG 1016): a randomised, multicentre, non-inferiority trial. Lancet. 2019;393(10166):40–50.
8. Mehanna H, Robinson M, Hartley A, et al. Radiotherapy plus cisplatin or cetuximab in low-risk human papillomavirus-positive oropharyngeal cancer (De-ESCALaTE HPV): an open-label randomized controlled phase 3 trial. Lancet. 2019 Jan;5(393):51–60.
9. Yom SS, Torres-Saavedra P, Caudell JJ, et al. Reduced-dose radiation therapy for HPV-associated oropharyngeal carcinoma (NRG Oncology HN002). J Clin Oncol. 2021;39(9):956–65.
10. https://www.nrgoncology.org/Clinical-Trials/Protocol/nrg-hn005?filter=nrg-hn005.
11. Ferris RL, Flamand Y, Weinstein GS, et al. Phase II randomized trial of transoral surgery and low-dose intensity modulated radiation therapy in resectable p16+ locally advanced oropharynx cancer: an ECOG-ACRIN cancer research group trial (E3311). J Clin Oncol. 2022;40(2):138–49.
12. Riaz N, Sherman E, Pei X, et al. Precision radiotherapy: reduction in radiation for oropharyngeal cancer in the 30 ROC trial. J Natl Cancer Inst. 2021;113(6):742–51.
13. Lee N, Sherman E, Schoder H, et al. Hypoxia-directed treatment of human papillomavirus-related oropharyngeal carcinoma. J Clin Oncol. 2023;42(8):940–50.
14. Ganly I, Goldstein D, Carlson DL, et al. Long-term regional control and survival in patients with "low-risk," early stage oral tongue cancer managed by partial glossectomy and neck dissection without postoperative radiation: the importance of tumor thickness. Cancer. 2013;119(6):1168–76.
15. Tian Q, Jiang L, Dai D, et al. Impact of postoperative radiotherapy on the progonosis of early-stage (pT1-2N0M0) oral tongue squamous cell carcinoma. J Clin Oncol. 2024;42(15):1754–65.
16. Bernier J, Domenge C, Ozsahin M, et al. European Organization for Research and Treatment of Cancer Trial 22931. Postoperative irradiation with or without concomitant chemotherapy for locally advanced head and neck cancer. N Engl J Med. 2004;350(19):1945–52.
17. Cooper JS, Pajak TF, Forastiere AA, et al. Radiation Therapy Oncology Group 9501/Intergroup. Postoperative concurrent radiotherapy and chemotherapy for high-risk squamous-cell carcinoma of the head and neck. N Engl J Med. 2004;350(19):1937–44.

18. Bernier J, Cooper JS, Pajak TF, et al. Defining risk levels in locally advanced head and neck cancers: a comparative analysis of concurrent postoperative radiation plus chemotherapy trials of the EORTC (#22931) and RTOG (# 9501). Head Neck. 2005 Oct;27(10):843–50.
19. Chen YP, Ismaila N, Chua MLK, et al. Chemotherapy in combination with radiotherapy for definitive-intent treatment of stage II-IVA nasopharyngeal carcinoma: CSCO and ASCO guideline. J Clin Oncol. 2021;39(7):840–59.
20. Chen QY, Wen YF, Guo L, et al. Concurrent chemoradiotherapy vs radiotherapy alone in stage II nasopharyngeal carcinoma: phase III randomized trial. J Natl Cancer Inst. 2011;103(23):1761–70.
21. Li XY, Chen QY, Sun XS, et al. Ten-year outcomes of survival and toxicity for a phase III randomised trial of concurrent chemoradiotherapy versus radiotherapy alone in stage II nasopharyngeal carcinoma. Eur J Cancer. 2019;110:24–31.
22. Al-Sarraf M, LeBlanc M, Giri PG, et al. Chemoradiotherapy versus radiotherapy in patients with advanced nasopharyngeal cancer: phase III randomized Intergroup study 0099. J Clin Oncol. 1998;16(4):1310–7.
23. Blanchard P, Lee A, Marguet S, et al. Chemotherapy and radiotherapy in nasopharyngeal carcinoma: an update of the MAC-NPC meta-analysis. Lancet Oncol. 2015;16(6):645–55.
24. Chen L, Hu CS, Chen XZ, et al. Concurrent chemoradiotherapy plus adjuvant chemotherapy versus concurrent chemoradiotherapy alone in patients with locoregionally advanced nasopharyngeal carcinoma: a phase 3 multicentre randomised controlled trial. Lancet Oncol. 2012;13(2):163–71.
25. Zhang Y, Chen L, Hu GQ, et al. Gemcitabine and cisplatin induction chemotherapy in nasopharyngeal carcinoma. N Engl J Med. 2019;381(12):1124–35.
26. Chen YP, Liu X, Zhou Q, et al. Metronomic capecitabine as adjuvant therapy in locoregionally advanced nasopharyngeal carcinoma: a multicentre, open-label, parallel-group, randomised, controlled, phase 3 trial. Lancet. 2021;398(10297):303–13.
27. https://www.nrgoncology.org/Clinical-Trials/Protocol/nrg-hn001?filter=nrg-hn001.
28. Mimica X, Yu Y, McGill M, et al. Organ preservation for patients with anterior mucosal squamous cell carcinoma of the nasal cavity: Rhinectomy-free survival in those refusing surgery. Head Neck. 2019 Aug;41(8):2741–7.
29. Yamazaki H, Nishiyama K, Tanaka E, et al. Radiotherapy for early glottic carcinoma (T1N0M0): results of prospective randomized study of radiation fraction size and overall treatment time. Int J Radiat Oncol Biol Phys. 2006;64(1):77–82.
30. Le Q-T, Fu K, Kroll S, et al. Influence of fraction size, total dose, and overall time on local control of T1-T2 glottic carcinoma. Int J Radiat Oncol Biol Phys. 1997;39(1):115–26.
31. Department of Veterans Affairs Laryngeal Cancer Study Group, Wolf GT, Fisher SG, et al. Induction chemotherapy plus radiation compared with surgery plus radiation in patients with advanced laryngeal cancer. N Engl J Med. 1991;324(24):1685–90.
32. Forastiere AA, Zhang Q, Weber RS, et al. Long-term results of RTOG 91-11: a comparison of three nonsurgical treatment strategies to preserve the larynx in patients with locally advanced larynx cancer. J Clin Oncol. 2013;31(7):845–52.
33. Eita A, Mohamed N, Rybkin A, et al. Outcomes for organ preservation with chemoradiation therapy for T4 larynx and hypopharynx cancer. Laryngoscope. 2022;133:1138.
34. Weber RS, Berkey BA, Forastiere A, et al. Outcome of salvage total laryngectomy following organ preservation therapy: the radiation therapy oncology group trial 91-11. Arch Otolaryngol Head Neck Surg. 2003;129(1):44–9.
35. Lefebvre JL, Andry G, Chevalier D, et al. Laryngeal preservation with induction chemotherapy for hypopharyngeal squamous cell carcinoma: 10-year results of EORTC trial 24891. Ann Oncol. 2012;23(10):2708–14.
36. Deschuymer S, Nevens D, Duprez F, et al. Randomized clinical trial on reduction of radiotherapy dose to the elective neck in head and neck squamous cell carcinoma; update of the long term tumor outcome. Radiother Oncol. 2020;143:24–9.

37. Deschuymer S, Nevens D, Duprez F, et al. Randomized clinical trial on reduction of radiotherapy dose to the elective neck in head and neck squamous cell carcinoma: results on the quality of life. Qual Life Res. 2021;30:117–27.
38. Tsai CJ, McBride SM, Riaz N, et al. Evaluation of substantial reduction in elective radiotherapy dose and field in patients with human papillomavirus-associated oropharyngeal carcinoma treated with definitive chemoradiotherapy. JAMA Oncol. 2022;8(3):364–72.
39. Lalla RV, Bowen J, Barasch A, et al. MASCC/ ISOO clinical practice guidelines for the management of mucositis secondary to cancer therapy. Cancer. 2014;120(10):1453–61.
40. Pappas PG, Kauffman CA, Andea DR, et al. Clinical practice guidelines for the management of candidiasis: 2016 update by the Infectious Diseases Society of America. Clin Infect Dis. 2016;62(4):e1–e50.

Lung Cancer

4

Annemarie Shepherd, Andreas Rimner, and Daniel Gomez

Lung cancer is the most common cause of cancer-related deaths. The majority of lung cancers are non-small cell lung cancer (NSCLC, 85%), and 15% are small cell lung cancers (SCLC). Early-stage NSCLC is generally treated with surgical resection or stereotactic body radiation therapy (SBRT). Locally advanced NSCLC is treated with a combination of modalities, which may include surgery, systemic therapy, and radiation therapy. Limited-stage SCLC is treated with concurrent chemotherapy and radiation therapy.

History and Workup

Essential components of the history and work-up for lung cancer include:

- Smoking history
- Pathology/histology (core biopsy/fine needle aspiration (FNA))
- Mutational status (e.g., EGFR, ALK, PD-L1)
- Surgery and Medical Oncology Assessments as needed
- Mediastinal staging (imaging vs. pathological)
- Comorbidities, particularly any history of interstitial lung disease or pulmonary fibrosis, as these patients are at high risk for radiation pneumonitis

A. Shepherd (✉) · D. Gomez
Radiation Oncology, Memorial Sloan Kettering Cancer Center, Basking Ridge, NJ, USA
e-mail: shephera@mskcc.org; gomezd@mskcc.org

A. Rimner
Department of Radiation Oncology, Medical Center – University of Freiburg, Faculty of Medicine, University of Freiburg, German Cancer Consortium (DKTK), Freiburg, Germany
e-mail: andreas.rimner@uniklinik-freiburg.de

J. J. Cuaron, L. Z. Braunstein (eds.), *Radiation Oncology Clinical Fundamentals*,
https://doi.org/10.1007/978-3-031-77559-8_4

Imaging

Key Components of the Imaging Workup Include:

- CT of the chest w/Contrast (contrast is encouraged to better visualize mediastinal lymph nodes as long as there is no contraindication to contrast, such as allergy or renal impairment)
- PET CT (within 6 weeks of simulation. If not, repeat PET scan)
- Brain MRI (optional for Stage I)

Stereotactic Body Radiation Therapy (SBRT)

Stereotactic Body Radiation Therapy (SBRT) is indicated in stage I NSCLC patients who are poor surgical candidates or who refuse surgery.

DOSES:

- Peripheral lesions: 18 Gy x 3 fractions or 34 Gy x 1 fraction
- Abutting chest wall: 12 Gy x 4 fractions
- Abutting diaphragm OR abutting the heart OR central tumor OR large tumor >3–5 cm (GTV within the No Fly Zone): 10 Gy x 5 fractions
- Abutting proximal airways, esophagus, compressing/invading the great vessels, or large tumor >5–7 cm: 7.5 Gy x 8 or 4 Gy x 15

SIMULATION:

- Thin-cut CT (2 mm)
- Arms up, Alpha Cradle, 4DCT. Isocenter at center of tumor.
  - For patients unable to bring 1 arm up, the contralateral arm down is OK.
  - For patients who have trouble bringing both arms up, treat arms down in Aquaplast. Make sure that the arms are snug by the side without an air gap between the arms and the torso.
  - Consider deep inspiratory breath hold (DIBH) for lesions at the level of the hilum or inferior lung. DIBH workflow consisting of 3 repetitive DIBH scans at simulation to verify reproducibility of DIBH, with a 4D simulation scan as backup.

CONTOURING:

- Normal structures: brachial plexus (as needed if within 4 slices of PTV), heart, carina, esophagus, proximal bronchial tree, No Fly zone (2 cm expansion of PBT), trachea (if tumor is in the upper lobes above the PBT; use same constraints at PBT), aorta and pulmonary artery, coronary arteries as indicated, 2 cm chest wall rind (4 slices above and below PTV), +/− liver, stomach, and kidney. See RTOG contouring atlas.

- Target Structures:
  - GTV
  - ITV (GTV + Motion)
  - CTV (2–3 mm expansion on ITV) can carve adjacent fixed structures (chest wall, great vessels, esophagus, PBT, heart) out of CTV if not invaded by tumor. CTV expansion is optional if treating pulmonary metastases
  - PTV = CTV + 3–5 mm

TREATMENT:

- OBI: CBCT each fraction matched to tumor.

Conventional Fractionation (Locally Advanced)

Definitive conventionally fractionated treatment is considered for patients with locally advanced NSCLC. Preoperative RT is typically not given at our institution, except in cases of Pancoast tumors

DOSES:

- Concurrent chemoradiation:
  - 60 Gy in 30 fractions
- Sequential chemotherapy or no chemotherapy:
  - 60–70 Gy, up to 70 Gy in 2 Gy/fraction
  - Or hypofractionation: 55 Gy in 20 Fraction or 60 Gy in 15 fractions depending on ability to meet OAR constraints
- Palliation: 600 cGy x 5 fractions, 300–400 cGy x 10–15 fractions

SIMULATION:

- PET/CT Sim, or fuse/refer to recent PET
- IV contrast to better evaluate mediastinal lymph nodes
- Arms up, Alpha Cradle, 4DCT. Isocenter at center of tumor.
  - For patients unable to bring 1 arm up, the contralateral arm down is OK.
  - For patients who have trouble bringing both arms up, treat arms down in Aquaplast.
  - Consider deep inspiratory breath hold (DIBH) for lesions at the level of the hilum or inferior lung.

CONTOURING:

- Normal structures: heart, carina, esophagus, +/− liver, kidney, stomach, brachial plexus
- GTV (PET avid or suspicious on CT, includes mediastinum)
- ITV (GTV + motion)

- CTV = ITV + 5–7 mm
  - Include the ipsilateral hilum
  - Try to connect in one volume if possible
  - Crop off critical structures
- PTV = CTV + 5 mm

TREATMENT:

- OBI: Daily KVs matched to bone (consider matching to carina for mediastinal/hilar targets if the discrepancy is too great between simulation and on- treatment images).
- Weekly CBCT to assess treatment response and the need for adaptive re-planning.

Post Operative Radiation Therapy

Post-operative radiation therapy (PORT) is considered for Stage III patients undergoing surgical resection with pathologically positive N2/N3 nodal disease, or positive margins (R1/R2 resection)

DOSES:

- Negative margins: 50.4 Gy in 28 fractions
- Positive margins: Dose paint to 54–60 Gy in 30 fractions
- Gross disease: Consider concurrent chemoradiation to 60 Gy in 30 fractions

SIMULATION:

- CT with IV contrast to better evaluate mediastinal nodal stations
- Arms up, Alpha Cradle, 4DCT. Isocenter at center of tumor.
  - For patients unable to bring 1 arm up, the contralateral arm down is OK.
  - For patients who have trouble bringing both arms up, treat arms down in Aquaplast. Make sure that the arms are snug by the side without an air gap between the arms and the torso.
  - Consider deep inspiratory breath hold (DIBH) for lesions at the level of the hilum or inferior lung. DIBH workflow consisting of 3 repetitive DIBH scans at simulation to verify reproducibility of DIBH, with a 4D simulation scan as backup.

CONTOURING:

- No GTV if R0-R1 resection
- CTV = involved nodal stations + bronchial stump + ipsilateral hilum
- ITV = CTV + respiratory motion
- PTV = ITV + 5 mm

TREATMENT:

- OBI: KVs each treatment (consider matching to carina for mediastinal/hilar targets if the discrepancy is too great between simulation and on- treatment images).
- Weekly CBCT to assess treatment response and the need for adaptive re-planning.

Small Cell Lung Cancer

Patients with limited-stage small cell lung cancer are treated with definitive concurrent chemoradiation therapy followed by PCI (consider use of memantine).

DOSES:

- 45 Gy in 1.5 Gy fractions delivered twice daily (BID)
- If BID is logistically infeasible for the patient, use 60–70 Gy in 30–35 fractions (see conventionally fractionated section above)

SIMULATION:

- PET/CT Sim, or fuse/refer to recent PET
- IV contrast to better evaluate mediastinal lymph nodes
- Arms up, Alpha Cradle, 4DCT. Isocenter at center of tumor
  - For patients unable to bring 1 arm up, the contralateral arm down is OK.
  - For patients who have trouble bringing both arms up, treat arms down in Aquaplast. Make sure that the arms are snug by the side without an air gap between the arms and the torso.
  - Consider deep inspiratory breath hold (DIBH) for lesions at the level of the hilum or inferior lung. DIBH workflow consisting of 3 repetitive DIBH scans at simulation to verify reproducibility of DIBH, with a 4D simulation scan as backup.

CONTOURING:

- Normal structures: heart, carina, esophagus, +/− liver, kidney, stomach, brachial plexus
- GTV (PET avid or suspicious on CT, includes mediastinum)
- ITV (GTV + motion)
- CTV = ITV + 5–7 mm
  - Include the ipsilateral hilum
  - Try to connect in one volume if possible
  - Crop off critical structures
- PTV = CTV + 5 mm

TREATMENT:

- OBI: KVs each treatment (consider matching to carina for mediastinal/hilar targets if the discrepancy is too great between simulation and on- treatment images).
- Weekly CBCT to assess treatment response and the need for adaptive re-planning.

Planning and Treatment Delivery

- Per MSK External Beam Guidelines

Ensure hot spots are not in the esophagus, proximal bronchial tree, or in vascular structures.

On Treatment Management and Follow-Up Care

Common toxicities

Acute:

- Cough: Robitussin→Tessalon→ Hycodan
- Esophagitis*: Diet modification→PPI→Carafate→Opiates, gabapentin, hydration/admission PRN
- *Consider fluconazole or nystatin for candidal esophagitis in DDx
- Dermatitis: Emollients→mometasone→silvadene
- Neutropenia: Hold RT for ANC <0.5. Resume once >0.5. Avoid G- CSF and GM-CSF except on a case-by-case basis with a medical oncologist.

Subacute:

- Pneumonitis (occurs 1–9 months after the completion of radiation): If clinically significant, start prednisone: 40 mg/day, then taper over 8–10 weeks contingent on symptoms. Include PPI and PCP Prophylaxis (Bactrim MWF).

Follow Up:

- Definitive RT (SBRT or conventionally fractionated): 3 months with chest CT (with or without contrast), then q3m thereafter for the first 2 years, then Q6 months until 5 years out, and then annually indefinitely.
- Locally advanced/BID: At 4–6 weeks for toxicity check (earlier if needed as symptoms tend to peak 1–2 weeks after the completion of radiation). Then, 3 months with chest CT with contrast, then q3m thereafter for the first 2 years, then Q6 months until 5 years out and then annually indefinitely.

- PORT: At 4–6 weeks for toxicity check (earlier if needed as symptoms tend to peak 1–2 weeks after the completion of radiation). Then, 6 months from surgery with chest CT with contrast, then q6m thereafter for the first 2 years, and then annually indefinitely.
- Further follow-up at discretion of physician.

Breast Cancer

5

Lior Z. Braunstein, Beryl McCormick, Simon N. Powell, and Atif J. Khan

History and Workup

- Age, family history, reproductive history, exposures, comorbidities
- Genetic screening for patients <50 years old with estrogen receptor positive (ER+) or < 60 years old with triple negative disease
- Contraindications to radiotherapy (RT):
  - Relative: prior RT (may be treated with repeat breast conservation per RTOG 1014) [1], active collagen vascular disease (especially scleroderma) because of risk for adverse cosmesis [2].
  - Absolute: *TP53* mutation, pregnancy
- Surgery: Mastectomy (modified radical, skin sparing, nipple sparing, immediate vs. delayed reconstruction), lumpectomy (re-excisions, concurrent mammoplastic reduction)
  - Immediate reconstruction is most common in our practice, with tissue expanders placed at the time of mastectomy. RT is typically delivered with expanders in place, and final implant exchange surgery takes place at least 6 months after RT completion. However, RT to the final implant is also acceptable, with similar overall cosmetic outcomes.
- Pathology: Size, multifocality/multicentricity, grade, margin status, hormone receptor status, HER2 status (IHC +/− FISH), lymphovascular invasion, OncotypeDX RS [3].
- Plans for systemic and hormonal therapy
  - Trastuzumab +/− pertuzumab may continue throughout RT

L. Z. Braunstein (✉) · B. McCormick · S. N. Powell · A. J. Khan
Department of Radiation Oncology, Memorial Sloan Kettering Cancer Center, New York, NY, USA
e-mail: BRAUNSTL@mskcc.org; mccormib@mskcc.org; powells@mskcc.org; khana7@mskcc.org

J. J. Cuaron, L. Z. Braunstein (eds.), *Radiation Oncology Clinical Fundamentals*,
https://doi.org/10.1007/978-3-031-77559-8_5

  - TDM-1 can be given during RT (for non-pCR HER2+ residual after neoadjuvant chemotherapy) [4]. Early data suggest the safety of this approach, although ongoing studies are collecting outcomes with concurrent therapy.
  - Capecitabine: prefer to complete RT prior to starting capecitabine due to synergistic effects and risk of toxicity. However, if giving concurrently, consider discussing a reduced dose with a medical oncologist (for TNBC residual after neoadjuvant chemotherapy); the dose was 1250 mg BID on CREATE-X; may consider concurrent therapy in the context of gross disease [5].
  - Palbociclib (and CDK4/6 inhibitors, generally) should be stopped for comprehensive RT; can continue cautiously for palliation.
  - Endocrine therapy may be initiated and continued throughout radiotherapy.
  - Pembrolizumab: prefer to hold until after radiotherapy but can be considered concurrently if needed (KEYNOTE 522) [6].

Imaging

- Review pre-operative mammogram, sonogram, MRI, PET
- Assess location of tumor and pre-therapy axillary, SCV, and IMN lymph node status
- Consider post-op mammo for DCIS with close margins
- Systemic staging (PET or CT CAP and bone scan) for: recurrent disease, 4+ nodes (N3+)

DCIS

- Indications for adjuvant radiotherapy (presence of any one of these factors is sufficient):
  - Presence of any grade 3 component on biopsy or surgery specimens
  - Size >2.5 cm
  - Age < 40
  - Any close margin (<2 mm). Note: if close margin is the sole indication for adjuvant RT, consider re-excision (discuss with the surgeon and patient)

    For patients undergoing RT, close (<2 mm) margins are not an absolute indication for re-excision (Tadros et al., Ann Surg 2019); it is okay to treat with close margins. Such cases should warrant discussion with the surgeon and patient.
- For all other risk factors and combinations of risk factors, discussion with the patient and the patient's risk tolerance for subsequent in-breast events needs to be discussed and considered. Observation can be considered for any patient not meeting the criteria above. Radiotherapy can be considered for any patient with DCIS, including low-risk/good-risk DCIS (depending on the risk tolerance of the patient). Approximate risk of total and invasive recurrence in the breast is:

	All/invasive events *without RT* (rounded to nearest integer)	All/invasive events *with RT* (rounded to nearest integer)
Low/int grade	15%/10% (15 years, 9804, 66% took endocrine therapy)	7%/5% (15 years, 9804, 58% took endocrine therapy)
High grade	25%/13% (12 years, ECOG 5194, 25% took tamoxifen)	3% (5 years, TROG07.01, high risk); 6–7% (10 years B39, all DCIS)

- Factors to consider include:
  - Definition of RTOG 9804: "Good Risk" (low or intermediate grade, < 2.5 cm, with margins >/= 3 mm) [7].
  - MSK nomogram risk
  - Age 40–50
  - ER status
  - Use of endocrine therapy
  - NOTE on size: In absence of frank measurement, one block is typically 3 mm thick, and a single slide is reviewed from each block. Approximate DCIS size = # positive slides × 3 mm.
- No PMRT for positive margin (according to Childs et al., IJROBP, 2013) but can bring to the breast team for discussion
- DCIS with microinvasion without axillary sampling: prefer whole breast RT
- +/− high tangents (avoid PBI)
- TECHNIQUE/DOSE:
- Hypofractionation (265 cGy × 16 fractions) to whole breast (TROG study).
- Consider PBI for any grade. DCIS if <3 cm (NSABP B39).
- (See below for PBI technique)
- Boost (if indicated, at discretion of treating MD): 235–250 cGy × 4.
- Note: A TROG randomized study demonstrated the benefit of boost in non-good-risk DCIS patients. Can omit for Good Risk.

SIMULATION:

- Supine, arms up on breast board.
- Deep inspiratory breath hold for left-sided cases.
- Consider PRONE for pendulous breast; however, for left sided tumor beds near the chest wall, supine DIBH often provides better cardiac sparing.

CONTOURING:

- Lumpectomy Boost: 2 cm expansion from cavity to block edge.
- Boost energy: Prescribed IDL should go all the way to the chest wall. Prescribed IDL measure skin to chest wall (E/3; i.e., 16MEV is ~5 cm depth to 90% IDL; 12MEV is ~4 cm).
- Use custom bolus as tissue compensation if tissue has variable thickness.

Early-Stage Node-Negative Disease

- MSK approach to elderly:
  - 75yo + pT1N0 →STRONGLY PREFER omission of RT if attempting hormonal therapy. Includes ER + HER2+ getting HER2-directed therapy.
  - 65–74yo → OK to omit if getting HT.If RT, then prefer PBI, or whole breast without boost.
- DEBRA Trial / NRG BR008) → pT1N0 ER+ 50–69yo, Oncotype<18; RCT RT vs obs
- FAST Forward (26Gy/5 daily): Can consider in 70yo+. If boost, 5.2Gy×1. No lower age limit for patients with travel issues and informed discussion of absence of >5yr outcomes.
- Boost is default when treating. Consider omission for:
  - Eligible for omission of RT (Khan maxim).
  - Also >60yo and gr1–2, no LVI, wide margin
- Consider PBI if eligible for omission but declines
- RNI should be rare for pT1–2 N0

DOSES for WBI:

- Hypofractionation (265 cGy × 16 fraction) to the whole breast.
- START B (267 cGy × 15 = 4005 cGy) is acceptable to finish in 3 weeks
- UK FAST FORWARD (5.2Gy × 5 = 26Gy in 1 week) for >80yo or poor KPS
- Boost (if indicated, see above): 250 cGy × 4

SIMULATION:

- Supine, arms up on breast board.
- Wires placed by therapists.
- Deep inspiratory breath hold for left-sided cases.
- Consider PRONE for pendulous breast; however, for left-sided tumor beds near the chest wall, supine DIBH often provides better cardiac sparing.

CONTOURING:

- Tangents and boosts designed in VSIM.
- Lumpectomy Boost:
  - 2 cm expansion from cavity to block edge
  - Boost energy: Prescribed IDL should go to the chest wall or 2 cm beyond the lumpectomy cavity. Prescribed IDL measure skin to chest wall (E/3; i.e., 16MEV is ~5 cm depth to 90% IDL; 12MEV is ~4 cm).
  - Electron Beam Data Tables available on Physics Team Share
  - Boost technique: For deep cavities, use a multi-beam photon arrangement with a PTV boost margin of 1 cm on the cavity. DO NOT use mini-tangents.

Pick a gantry angle that is perpendicular to the CW for most patients. However, for superficial lumpectomy cavities, perpendicular to the skin is preferred.
- Use custom bolus as tissue compensation if tissue has variable thickness.

Partial Breast Irradiation

Can be offered for patients meeting ASTRO “suitable” or “cautionary” criteria.

- Risk factors include: 2–3 cm, focal LVI (not including LVI NOS or extensive), lobular, ER-, EIC (can discuss with pathologist), and margin <2 mm.
  - 40–49yo with no risk factors
  - 50–65yo + with up to 1 risk factor
  - 66yo + with up to 2 risk factors
- At MSK, unsuitable: age < 40, positive margin, any tumor >3 cm (invasive or DCIS any grade), extensive LVI, germline BRCA, and ATM mutation carriers; **for oncotype > 26, prefer whole breast or PBI**.

DOSES for PBI:

- 400 × 10 delivered every day for 2 weeks. 30Gy/5# allowed; CONTOURING: (http://econtour.org/cases/108).
- Contour whole breast, cavity, heart, nipple, and surgical clips.
- Margins: Lumpectomy cavity + 1.5–2.0 cm to CTV + 0.5 cm to PTV (can shrink CTV expansion to 1 cm for a large seroma).
- CTV should be limited anteriorly to exclude 5 mm below the skin surface and posteriorly to exclude the pectoralis muscles, ribs, and chest wall structures.
- The PTV should be a uniform expansion for aperture generation.
- PTV_DVH will be limited anteriorly to within 5 mm below the skin surface.
- PTV should not exceed 25–30% of whole breast volume (=PTV/whole breast); <25% acceptable, <30% limit

TREATMENT:

Daily KVs matched to clips; if no clips and close to CW, consider CBCT match to ribs

Upfront Surgery, Node-Positive

NODAL STAGING:

- Isolated tumor cells (ITCs) or < 0.2 mm positive on IHC are pN0(i+).
- Intramammary nodes are pN1.
- Micrometastases (≤2 mm) → pN1mi → no nodal RT in general (“Cahlon’s 99% rule”) unless 3 or more nodes (see Risk Matrix).

POST LUMPECTOMY RT:

- High tangents (covering levels I and II of the axilla) acceptable for 1–2 positive SLN macromets (>2 mm) in low-risk patients (age > 50, T1–2, no LVI, ER + Her2-, low oncotype, no extranodal extension) per ACOSOG Z0011.

Consider regional nodal RT for patients meeting criteria per Risk Matrix (below).
POST MASTECTOMY RT (PMRT):

- Consider adjuvant regional nodal irradiation depending on concomitant risk factors. For patients undergoing breast conservation or for those undergoing mastectomy with axillary lymph node dissection, we consider the following in deciding upon regional nodal irradiation:
  - Primary risk factors include age <40, triple negative disease, and the presence of extensive lymphovascular invasion or tumor emboli in axillary soft tissue.
  - Secondary risk factors to consider include: high grade, medial location, tumor >3 cm, high Oncotype DX recurrence score, age 40–50, lymphovascular invasion, extracapsular extension.
  - For patients who are **node-negative**, we consider regional nodal irradiation if all 3 primary and 1 secondary risk factor are present, or if only 2 primary and 3 secondary risk factors are present.
  - For patients with a **single positive node**, we consider regional nodal irradiation if there is evidence of extensive LVI, if the patient is <40 years old with TNBC, if LVI is present with at least one secondary risk factor, or if 3 secondary risk factors are present.
  - For patients with **two positive nodes**, we consider regional nodal irradiation if any primary risk factor is present, or if the patient exhibits LVI, or if the patient is 40–50 years of age, or if any 2 secondary risk factors are present.
  - For patients with **three or more positive nodes**, we routinely recommend regional nodal irradiation.
- Of note, the above considerations refer to those receiving upfront surgery.
- Generally, any patient with ypN+, yp(ITC), or ypN0 but clinically N+ disease requires RNI/PMRT. NSABP B-51 is evaluating the possibility of de-escalating this approach.
- Mastectomy pts. with SNBx only and any macromets require PMRT or go back to the OR for ALND.
- See surgical risk table for decision rule on combinations of age <40 and TNBC with degree of nodal involvement as indications for RNI/PMR. These patients may not have had ALND but meet criteria for PMRT.
- For combinations of micro and macrometases, generally consider the micromet to be an additional +node. Consider the difficult case discussion.

If the patient is known to meet criteria for RT intraoperatively based on a combination of these factors (e.g., 2+ nodes, age 45–50, medial tumor), ALND will not be performed provided that <3+ nodes are present.

- For patients with 3 or more nodes involved with micromets and/or ITCs, consider using the "2+ nodes" to determine indication for RNI (or MD discretion, present to the breast team).
- For pT3N0 cases: Default is PMRT but consider omitting PMRT for >60y, <7 cm, no LVI (See below "NAC" for cT3N0)

DOSES:

- Lumpectomy, no RNI: 265 cGy × 16 + Boost (235–250 cGy × 4 sequential).
- Lumpectomy with RNI: 200 × 25 + sequential boost (200 x 5) or simultaneous integrated boost (230–240 cGy × 25).
  - NOTE: Margin on GTV should be smaller for SIB.
  - (0.7–1.5 cm to final boost PTV); remember, 230 cGy is EQD2 60Gy
- PMRT: 200 × 25.
  - If flat chest wall, can consider 42.56 in 16 for flat chest wall (esp older patient).
  - If reconstruction, enroll on RT CHARM (18–476).
- Scar boost sequential 200 × 5.
- Node boost.
  - Gross residual: sequential (200 x 6–8) vs. SIB (240 cGy × 25).
  - Unresected nodes that have responded to chemo: sequential (200 × 5) or SIB (225 × 25).
  - NOTE: sequentially preferred abutting brachial plexus (if SIB, max 225 cGy/Fx).

Other Planning Considerations:

- CW alone (without RNI) only for select positive margin cases (to be used rarely).

Scar boost: for recurrent disease (but can omit if re-RT); can consider for skin involvement (T4b), N3+, positive margins, problem not for inflammatory disease (Damast et al. used 1 cm bolus daily).

Bolus Guidelines

	Clinical situation	Tangent fields, 6MVX	Tangent fields, 15MVX (Only used in case of tissue expander and/or for center breast ≥25 cm[a] at posterior border)	IMRT/ VMAT, 6MVX
Basic physics bolus	**Intact breast**	–	3 mm daily	3 mm daily[b,c]
	Tissue expander	–(Do not use 6MVX tangents)	1 cm daily	3 mm daily
	Mastectomy (with or without prosthesis)	3 mm daily	1 cm daily	3 mm daily
MD discretion	**High risk intact breast**	3 mm daily	5 mm daily	3 mm daily
	High risk of skin involvement (PMRT)	5 mm daily	1.3 cm daily	5 mm daily
	Inflammatory	1 cm daily	1.5 cm daily	1 cm daily

[a]If high energy machine is easily available, can consider >23 cm
[b]Due to enface beam dose contribution and acting as skin flash
[c]MD can choose not to use 3 mm bolus based on clinical judgement (planner should confirm before planning)

Skin Dose Requirements:

Skin Inside GTV (Inflammatory): ≥ 100% Rx Dose
Skin Inside GTV (High Risk of skin Involvement): At least 90% to 95% Rx Dose
Skin Inside CTV (Mastectomy): At least 85% to 90% Rx Dose
Skin Outside CTV (Intact Breast): At least 70% to 80% Rx Dose

Recommend to start with the amount using guideline, reduce or remove bolus amount later based on clinical assessment

SIMULATION:

- Supine, arms up, breast board
- Wires placed by therapists
- DIBH for left-sided cases TECHNIQUE (3D vs. IMRT)
- Use of IMRT/VMAT vs. 3DCRT is case-dependent. IMRT provides for a more homogenous dose distribution and superior coverage of target at the expense of increased low-dose bath to the cardiopulmonary structures.
- Relative indications for VMAT include:
  - High-risk patients needing complete coverage of full axilla and IMNs
  - High-riding contralateral implant precluding coverage of IMNs with tangents
  - Inability to both target IMNs and meet lung or heart constraints due to patient anatomy

CONTOURING:

- RADCOMP contouring atlas and MSKCC patterns of failure atlas [8]
  - SCV should be contoured to the posterior edge of the middle scalene. "Posterior neck" extends to the trapezius and should be used for high-risk patients.
- Contour CTV_Axilla, CTV_SCLAV, CTV_IMN, and CTV_chest wall and breast
- Boolean chest wall/breast with axilla/sclav/IMN into CTV50

Expand CTV50 by 0.5 mm for PTV50. Hand edit PTV50 as needed.

Inflammatory Breast Cancer

- Mastectomy, ALND, PMRT for all, prefer delayed reconstruction.
- DOSE same as PMRT except:
  - Scar boost (10Gy/5) is optional because use daily CW bolus (per Damast IJROBP 2010)
- CONTOURING same as PMRT, except:
  - Always include posterior neck
  - Scar boost (if included, though not mandatory, per above): 2 cm margin on mastectomy scar
- RX:
- CW Bolus 1 cm and keep throughout treatment (regardless of skin reaction). Use a 1.5 cm bolus for 15 MV plans.

Reirradiation

Favor treating partial breast [9] (per RTOG 1014)

Favor avoiding re-RT to brachial plexus. If needed, keep cumulative maximum dose to plexus ~75–78 Gy.

Refer to the upfront decision matrix above, but consider extensive multidisciplinary review

DOSES: PBI: 45Gy/25 (MSK preferred) [9] or 45Gy/30 BID (RTOG 1014)

Palliative Regimens

Suggested regimens for palliative breast radiotherapy for patients with metastatic or gross unresectable disease.

- Favor treating whole breast rather than partial breast
- Short course
  - 27–30Gy/5fx
  - Can also consider 30Gy/10fx (though note lower BED)
  - Consider boosting gross disease; 7Gy × 5 with simultaneous integrated boost (SIB) or 6Gy × 6
- Intermediate course.
  - 37.5–45Gy/15fx (favored schedule if treating RNI)
  - Consider boosting gross disease to 52.5Gy SIB or sequential 10Gy/4.

Plan Review

- Review cross-sectional images to ensure adequate coverage of the breast/chest wall and all nodal areas
- IMN coverage >80% isodose line (i.e., 40 Gy for a conventionally-fractionated 50Gy prescription) for low risk
- For VMAT plans, aim for mean heart dose ideal <4 Gy, acceptable 5 Gy

References

1. Arthur DW, Winter KA, Kuerer HM, et al. Effectiveness of breast-conserving surgery and 3-dimensional conformal partial breast reirradiation for recurrence of breast cancer in the ipsilateral breast: the NRG oncology/RTOG 1014 phase 2 clinical trial. JAMA Oncol. 2020;6(1):75–82.
2. Wo J, Taghian A. Radiotherapy in setting of collagen vascular disease. Int J Radiat Oncol Biol Phys. 2007;69(5):1347–53.
3. Braunstein LZ, Taghian AG, Niemierko A, et al. Breast-cancer subtype, age, and lymph node status as predictors of local recurrence following breast-conserving therapy. Breast Cancer Res Treat. 2017;161:173–9.
4. Von Minckwitz G, Huang C-S, Mano MS, et al. Trastuzumab emtansine for residual invasive HER2-positive breast cancer. N Engl J Med. 2019;380(7):617–28.
5. Mayer IA, Zhao F, Arteaga CL, et al. Randomized phase III postoperative trial of platinum-based chemotherapy versus capecitabine in patients with residual triple-negative breast cancer following neoadjuvant chemotherapy: ECOG-ACRIN EA1131. J Clin Oncol. 2021;39(23):2539.

6. Schmid P, Cortes J, Pusztai L, et al. Pembrolizumab for early triple-negative breast cancer. N Engl J Med. 2020;382(9):810–21.
7. McCormick B, Moughan J, Hudis C, et al. Low-risk breast ductal carcinoma in situ (DCIS): results from the Radiation Therapy Oncology Group 9804 phase 3 trial. Int J Radiat Oncol Biol Phys. 2012;84(3):S5.
8. DeSelm C, Yang TJ, Cahlon O, et al. A 3-dimensional mapping analysis of regional nodal recurrences in breast cancer. Int J Radiat Oncol Biol Phys. 2019;103(3):583–91.
9. Chen I, Botty Van den Bruele AM, Gillespie EF, et al. Salvage of locally recurrent breast cancer with repeat breast conservation using 45 Gy hyperfractionated partial breast re-irradiation. Breast Cancer Res Treat. 2021;188:409–14.

Gastrointestinal Cancers

6

Marsha Reyngold, Carla Hajj, Abraham Wu, Paul Romesser, and Chris Crane

Esophagus and GE Junction

Neoadjuvant chemoradiotherapy (CRT) followed by surgery is the standard approach for patients with locally advanced squamous cell carcinoma (SCC) and some patients with adenocarcinoma (AC). Organ preservation approaches for SCC can be considered on a case-by-case basis for patients treated with definitive intent. For patients with locally advanced adenocarcinoma, CRT or perioperative chemotherapy can be considered in consultation with the disease management team (DMT). Induction chemotherapy followed by PET response-adapted CRT is favored at MSK for PET-avid adenocarcinomas. For patients who are not surgical candidates, CRT is the default option.

History and Workup

- Surgical candidacy
- Adenocarcinoma vs. squamous cell carcinoma
- Siewert Classification (Siewert I/II: Esophagus paradigm; Siewert III: Esophagus or Stomach paradigm)
- GEJ tumor: consider staging laparotomy (for Siewert III)

M. Reyngold (✉) · A. Wu · P. Romesser · C. Crane
Department of Radiation Oncology, Memorial Sloan Kettering Cancer Center, New York, NY, USA
e-mail: reyngolM@mskcc.org; wua@mskcc.org; romessep@mskcc.org; cranec1@mskcc.org

C. Hajj
Oncology Institute, Cleveland Clinic Abu Dhabi, Abu Dhabi, United Arab Emirates
e-mail: Hajjc@clevelandclinicabudhabi.ae

J. J. Cuaron, L. Z. Braunstein (eds.), *Radiation Oncology Clinical Fundamentals*,
https://doi.org/10.1007/978-3-031-77559-8_6

- Tumors suspected of invading trachea: bronchoscopy

Imaging

- Esophagus: PET/CT and CT CAP with contrast

Planning and Treatment Delivery

- Adenocarcinoma: Induction FOLFOX PET assessment FOLFOX/CapeOx-based CRT for SUV change ≥35% or carboplatin/paclitaxel-based CRT (SUV change <35%) per CALGB 80803
- Alternative chemotherapy: carboplatin/paclitaxel
- No role for induction chemotherapy with PET negative (SUV <5)
- SCC: Concurrent chemoradiation with weekly carboplatin/ paclitaxel
- IMRT preferred over 3D-CRT to spare heart and lungs
- Role of protons is being investigated in an RCT (NRG GI006)—enrollment on trial preferred

DOSES:

- Thoracic/abdominal esophageal CA: 50.4 Gy in 1.8 Gy fractions (pre-op or definitive)
- Alternatives:
  - 45 Gy if significant gastric involvement
  - 41.4 Gy +/− cone-down to 45 Gy if volume is very large and not meeting OAR constraints.
- Cervical esophageal CA: typically 54/60 Gy in 27–30 fractions with dose-painting IMRT to PTV gross disease and 45–50 Gy to areas at risk for microscopic spread
- No role for further dose escalation beyond what is outlined above

SIMULATION:

- Consider fiducial placement and respiratory gating for GEJ tumors
- NPO (2–3 hours prior to simulation or treatments)
- Thoracic/abdominal esophageal CA: Arms up, alpha cradle, 4D-CT, IV contrast (PO barium immediately prior to scan is optional)
- Cervical esophageal CA: Arms down, 7-point mask, IV contrast
- Isocenter: center of GTV

CONTOURING:

- Contour normal structures

  - Esophagus
  - Stomach
  - Small bowel and large bowel were near field
  - Brachial plexus, if applicable
  - Heart
  - Lungs
- Contour GTV based on PET and cross-reference with EGD findings (entire lumen circumference is included at involved levels)
- Reference: Wu AJ Et al. Expert Consensus Contouring Guidelines for Intensity Modulated Radiation Therapy in Esophageal and Gastroesophageal Junction Cancer. Int J Radiation Oncol Biol Phys. 2015;92:911–920

On Treatment Management and Follow-Up Care

COMMON TOXICITIES:

- Nausea/Vomiting: pretreatment anti-emetics, PPI
- Esophagitis: Diet modification→PPI → Carafate→Opiates
- Neutropenia: Hold RT for ANC <1.0. Resume once >1.0
- Thrombocytopenia: Hold RT for platelets <50

FOLLOW-UP SCHEDULE:

- 4 weeks post RT: Rad Onc Tox Check, PET/CT and CT CAP, CBC, surgical evaluation +/− endoscopy as appropriate
- Follow q3-month with CT and blood work

Gastric Cancer

For patients with gastric cancer, RT is used primarily for palliation, definitive therapy for medically inoperable patients, and for select patients after a resection. RT has been largely supplanted by peri-operative chemotherapy for most patients with locally advanced Siewert III GEJ and gastric cancers due to a more favorable toxicity profile of the latter and lower chance of R1 resection compared to esophageal cancers.

History and Workup

- Surgical candidacy
- Staging laparoscopy

Imaging

- CT CAP with contrast and PET/CT

Planning and Treatment Delivery

- Post-op for positive margins after resection
- Definitive therapy for medically inoperable patients with locally advanced disease
- Palliation of bleeding tumors

DOSES:

- Post-op or definitive: 45 Gy in 1.8 Gy per fraction boost to 50.4 Gy
- Palliative regimens: 35 Gy in 2.5 Gy per fraction, 30 Gy in 3.0 Gy per fraction, or 20 Gy in 4 Gy per fraction

SIMULATION:

- NPO (2–3 hours prior to simulation and treatments)
- Arms up, alpha cradle, 4D-CT, IV contrast

CONTOURING:

- No established standard. Guides for post-op (+/− definitive) include:
  - CRITICS Trial protocol documents
  - MacDonald Trial methods
  - NCCN Guidelines
  - Wo JY et al. Gastric lymph node contouring atlas: A tool to aid in clinical target volume definition in 3-dimensional treatment planning for gastric cancer. Pract Radiat Oncol. 2013 Jan-Mar;3(1):e11–e19

On Treatment Management and Follow-Up Care

COMMON TOXICITIES:

- Nausea/Vomiting: pretreatment anti-emetics, PPI
- Monitor weight, PO intake
- Esophagitis: Diet modification→PPI → Carafate→Opiates
- Neutropenia: Hold RT for ANC <1.0. Resume once >1.0
- Thrombocytopenia: Hold RT for platelets <50

FOLLOW-UP SCHEDULE:

Based on goals of care, q3-month imaging, CBC, and symptom review if appropriate

Pancreatic Cancer

The role for RT in the management of pancreatic cancer has remained very controversial due to inconsistent findings from clinical trials, further complicated by evolving chemotherapy standards and the use of RT doses likely too low for a radioresistant histology. Several trials evaluating RT in the neoadjuvant/adjuvant setting are ongoing. In the definitive setting, dose escalation has been embraced at several institutions based on compelling retrospective evidence alone.

At MSK, for patients with borderline resectable disease, RT can be considered for those who continue to have vessel involvement after induction chemotherapy. Post-op RT is offered for patients with R1-resected disease and can be considered for select patients with other high-risk features. For cases where doses ≤50 Gy in 25–28 fractions are considered, IMRT or 3D-CRT can be used depending on individual anatomy and OARs.

For patients with locally advanced or locally recurrent disease, ablative approaches with dose escalation to >98Gy BED with either IMRT with motion management, CBCT-guidance and selective adaptive re-planning or MRgRT with daily adaptive replanning are preferred.

History and Workup

- Resectability and surgical candidacy
- CA 19–9

Imaging

- Pancreas: CT Angio Pancreas with chest/pelvis

Planning and Treatment Delivery

DOSES:

- **PRE-OP (BORDERLINE):** 36 Gy in 12–15 fractions (3D-CRT preferred for expediency/cost effectiveness: IMRT is useful for cases with a significant amount of small bowel in the field).
- **DEFINITIVE (LAPC or isolated local recurrence after prior surgery):** Two dose levels using simultaneous integrated boost, $PTV_{\text{high-dose}}$ and $PTV_{\text{microscopic dose.}}$

- 67.5/37.5 Gy in 15 fractions or 75/45 Gy in 25 fractions (IMRT, motion management, CBCT-guidance required). 25-fraction regimen preferred for direct abutment of GTV with luminal GI organs at risk
- 50/33 Gy in 5 fractions (MRgRT only)

- **POST-OP (CLOSE or POS margins, N0 or low LN ratio):**
  - For adjuvant RT including R0 and R1 cases limited to retroperitoneal margin or other margins not anastamosed or adjacent tomucosa, use a 15-fraction regimen—microscopic dose of 37.5 Gy and + margin dose of 60 Gy if normal tissue constraints allow. Otherwise, use 45 and 65Gy in 25 fractions for microscopic and + margin volumes, respectively. Contours per Ablative Dosing below.
  - For unfavorable anatomy/mucosa-based margin, use 54 Gy in 27 fractions IMRT. Contours per RTOG Atlas.
- **PALLIATIVE:**
  - 30Gy/10 fractions preferred
  - 20Gy/5 or 36 Gy/15 fractions acceptable depending on clinical situation.

SIMULATION:

- NPO 2–3 hours prior to simulation and treatment
- 3D-CRT or conventional-dose IMRT:
  - Alpha cradle, arms up, 4D-CT optional (will require larger margins if not used), IV contrast optional
  - Isocenter at GTV
- Ablative dosing (hypofractionated IMRT):
  - Require metal stents or fiducials
  - Alpha cradle, arms up (if no shoulder problems)
  - Motion management: DIBH simulation CT preferred, gated 4D-CT for patients who can't comply. If gated treatment is not possible, an ITV approach in a free-breathing patient can be considered on a case-by-case basis only.
  - IV contrast pancreatic protocol: 150 cc at 5 cc/sec, requires at least 20-gauge IV, timing of scan after injection depends on motion management technique
    DIBH: 45 sec and 1.5 min delay from start of injection
    4D-CT: start both at the same time
  - Isocenter at GTV
- Ablative dosing (MRgRT):
  - Arms down, CT and MR simulation scans
  - Motion management: compression belt
  - IV contrast-enhanced (unless contraindicated) pancreatic protocol CT: 150 cc at 5 cc/sec 45 sec delay
  - IV contrast-enhanced (unless contraindicated) MRI

– Isocenter at GTV

CONTOURING:

- **3D-CRT OR CONVENTIONAL-DOSE IMRT FOR PRE-OP:**

Target volumes	Definition and description
GTV	All gross disease on imaging, including the primary tumor (typically hypointense), paying particular attention to extension along the vessels (including entire vessel circumference at the level of the tumor), and all suspicious nodes
ITV-optional	If using the ITV approach, use the guideline for GTV delineation on all phases of the 4D-CT
CTV	Given the infiltrative nature of PDAC, adequate margin is critical and should include at least 1 cm uniform expansion on all gross disease. + coverage of CA and SMA basins + coverage of Para-aortic basins at the level of GTV up to the anterior surface of the bone posteriorly + additional margin along vessels if there is any uncertainty regarding tumor extension
PTV	PTV margin is based on the motion management technique used (if any) and should be at least 0.5 cm. For cases treated with FB and without an ITV, expansions of ≥1.5 cm in the superior-inferior dimension are recommended

OARs: stomach, small bowel, large bowel, kidneys, liver, spinal cord

- **CONVENTIONAL-DOSE (IMRT FOR POST-OP)**
  – The RTOG 0848 contouring atlas provides a stepwise contouring approach based on identifiable regions of interest (ROI) that were chosen on the basis of ease of identification and reproducibility in imaging studies. However, smaller fields targeting the postoperative bed, CA, and SMA only may be appropriate in clinical scenarios with dose-limiting OARs.
- **ABLATIVE DOSING (DEFINITIVE FOR POST-OP)**
  – Dose-painting is used to shape hot spots and microscopic dose clouds—MULTIPLE PTVs.
  – All high-dose PTVs must exclude the GI tract with additional safety margin.
  – Planning requires PRVs for all luminal OARs.
  – **HYPOFRACTIONATED IMRT:**

Target volumes	Definition and description
GTV	All gross disease on imaging, including the primary tumor (typically hypointense), paying particular attention to extension along the vessels (including entire vessel circumference at the level of the tumor), and all suspicious nodes
ITV-optional	If using the ITV approach, use the guidelines for GTV delineation on all phases of the 4D-CT
$CTV_{high\ dose}$	Corresponds to GTV or ITV if used without additional margin
$CTV_{microscopic\ dose}$	Given the infiltrative nature of PDAC, adequate margin is critical and should include the following. Areas at risk are defined by the location of nodal basins but are also meant to cover the perineural networks within those regions. 1 cm uniform expansion on all gross disease (to ensure coverage of peripancreatic nodes). + coverage of CA and SMA basins + coverage of Para-aortic basins at the level of GTV up to the anterior surface of the bone posteriorly + splenic hilum basin (body/tail lesions only) + additional margin along vessels if there is any uncertainty regarding tumor extension (e.g., CHA for tumors involving the CA) Optional: Coverage of the porta hepatis basin (for head of the pancreas tumors)
$PTV_{high\ dose}$	Uniform expansion $CTV_{high\ dose}$ by 0.5 cm followed by subtraction of any overlapping critical OAR (stomach, small bowel, large bowel) with additional safety margin of 0.5 cm. Alternative: a 0.7 cm safety margin should be used if there is a significant interface between the target and the given OAR)
$PTV_{microscopic\ dose}$	PTV margin is based on the motion management technique used (if any) and should be at least 0.5 cm. No subtraction of OARs is used here.
Notable OAR volumes	Applicable for doses ≥60Gy in 25 fractions (or BED equivalent)
Stomach-Proximal Duodenum PRV	Stomach and duodenum segments 1 and 2 + 3–5 mm
Small Bowel PRV	All other small bowel +3–5 mm
Bile Duct PRV	Bile duct from CBD to and including the second-order bile ducts (e.g., right and left hepatic ducts) + 5 mm. Alternative: Can use PV as a surrogate for bile duct location +10 mm

– **MRgRT**

Target volumes	Definition and Description
GTV	As above
$CTV_{high\ dose}$	As above
$CTV_{microscopic\ dose}$	As above
$PTV_{high\ dose}$	Uniform expansion of GTV=$CTV_{high\ dose}$ by 0.5 cm followed by subtraction of any overlapping critical OAR (stomach, small bowel, large bowel) with additional safety margin of 0.3 cm.
$PTV_{microscopic\ dose}$	Uniform expansion of $CTV_{microscopic\ dose}$ by 0.5 cm followed by subtraction of any overlapping critical OAR (stomach, small bowel, large bowel) without any additional safety margin.
Notable OAR volumes	Applicable for doses ≥60Gy in 25 fractions (or BED equivalent)

(continued)

Target volumes	Definition and Description
Stomach-Proximal Duodenum PRV	Stomach and duodenum segments 1 and 2 + 1 mm
Small Bowel PRV	All other small bowel +1 mm
Bile Duct PRV	Bile duct from CBD to and including the second-order bile ducts (e.g., right and left hepatic ducts) + 1 mm.

On Treatment Management and Follow-Up Care

COMMON TOXICITIES:

- Nausea/Vomiting: pretreatment anti-emetics (mandatory for MRgRT, otherwise optional), PPI.
- Imodium and lorazepam are administered for MRgRT patients on days of treatment to reduce bowel motion and patient movement.
- Esophagitis: Diet modification→PPI → Carafate→Opiates.
- Diarrhea: Low fat, low fiber diet modification ➔ Imodium → Lomotil → Tincture of Opium → Chemo dose adjustment or discontinuation → RT break.
- Neutropenia: Hold RT for ANC <1.0. Resume once >1.0.

FOLLOW-UP SCHEDULE:

- 6–8 weeks post RT: Rad Onc Tox Check, CT Angio Pancreas w/ Chest and Pelvis, CBC, Ca19–9 (CEA for non-secretors)
- Follow q3m with CT and blood work

Liver and Liver Metastases

Experience with external beam radiation therapy for the treatment of hepatocellular carcinoma (HCC) and liver metastases has been rapidly built over the past 2 decades, enabled and accelerated by advanced technologies such as IMRT, SBRT, and proton therapy. There is a smaller, albeit no less encouraging experience with intrahepatic cholangiocarcinoma (IHCC). Proton therapy has been extensively used for HCC outside of the US and is hypothesized to reduce the chance of liver decompensation in patients with liver disease. At MSKCC, outside of the clinical trial comparing protons to photons (NRG-GI003), we consider proton therapy for patients with large liver tumors. With regard to liver metastases, dose escalation beyond 100Gy BED may be needed for more radioresistant histologies.

History and Workup

- LFTs

- Child-Pugh score for patients with cirrhosis (Bilirubin, Albumin, PT/INR, Ascites, Encephalopathy)
  - Albumin: >35 g/l = 1 point; 28–35 g/l = 2 points; <28 g/l = 3 points
  - Bilirubin: <2 mg/dl = 1 point; 2–3 mg/dl = 2 points; >3 mg/ dl = 3 points
  - Prothrombrin INR: 1 point if <1.7; 2 points if 1.7–2.3; 3 points if >2.3
  - Ascites*: absent = 1 point; mild = 2 points; marked (moderate-to-severe) = 3 points
  - Hepatic encephalopathy: 1 point if none; 2 points if mild (grade I–II, or responsive to medication); 3 points if marked (grade III–IV, or refractory to treatment)
  - Consider RT for CP A and B7 only
- HCC/IHCC: Number of liver nodules and their size, extrahepatic spread, vascular invasion/tumor vessel thrombus (TVT), presence of portal hypertension
- Metastasis: KPS, systemic disease status, tumor histology, symptomatic vs. not, number, location, and size of lesions, other treatments (particularly hepatic artery infusion pump chemotherapy and radioembolization, or Y90)

Imaging

- 3 phase CT (4 phase CT for HCC) (Eovist enhanced MRI for small lesions that cannot be classified by CT)

Planning and Treatment Delivery

More stringent liver constraints are used for primary liver tumors, history of cirrhosis, or patients with HAI pumps. Prior Y90 therapy may require exclusion of segments treated with Y90 from healthy liver OAR used for optimization.

DOSES:

- **PRIMARY LIVER TUMORS:**
- HCC, IHCC, select hilar cholangiocarcinoma:
  - Two dose levels using simultaneous integrated boost, $PTV_{high\text{-}dose}$ and $PTV_{microscopic\ dose}$.
  - >1 cm from stomach/small bowel and meeting liver constraints:

67.5Gy/37.5Gy in 15 fractions (BED_{10} 98Gy) or 50–60/30Gy in 5 fractions (BED_{10} 100Gy)

All others: 75/45Gy in 25 fractions (BED_{10} 98Gy)

Lower doses may be considered for HCC to meet liver constraints

Strongly consider protons for large HCC and/or Child Pugh score of ≥ B7

- **METASTASIS:**
- For patients with good functional status, limited disease, and a reasonable life expectancy, they NEED to deliver **>95Gy BED_{10}**

- Two dose levels using simultaneous integrated boost, $PTV_{high\text{-}dose}$ and $PTV_{microscopic\ dose}$.

  60Gy/30Gy in 5 or 6 fractions (BED10 120–132) for lesions <6 cm in size AND > 2 cm from stomach/small bowel AND > 1 cm from large bowel

  If central (i.e., PTV involving bile ducts), abutting the chest wall and/or diaphragm 50/30Gy in 5 fractions or more fractionated approaches are preferred

  ALTERNATIVE if not meeting constraints (listed in the order of least to most sparing for normal tissue OARs):

  - 60–70/32Gy in 10 fractions (BED10 96–119)
  - 67.5/37.5Gy in 15 fractions (BED10 98)
  - 75/45Gy in 25 fractions (BED10 98)

  ALTERNATIVE acceptable for small peripheral lesions (>2 cm of PV bifurcation) 60/21Gy in 3 fractions (BED10 112–180)

Lower palliative dosing can be used for patients with poor functional status, widespread disease, or limited life expectancy at the discretion of the physician.

SIMULATION:

- NPO 2–3 hrs
- Consider the need for fiducials as in the motion management section and refer to IR if needed
  - Surgical clips or metal stents within close vicinity of the gross disease may be used instead
- Motion Management Order of Preference:

DIBH >	**CATING >**	**FREE BREATHING**
(Match on Fiducials or liver shape)	(Match on Fiducials	(Match on bone)

- Deep inspiration breath hold CT preferred (set up to fiducial (preferred) or liver shape if no fiducials AND tumor in the right hepatic lobe or seg 4A-B).
- Fiducial is needed if in the mobile left lobe of the liver (seg 2–3).
- Respiratory gating using Varian RPM for patients unable to comply with DIBH (requires fiducials).
- 4D CT (set up to bone) as the absolute last resort for patients unable to comply with DIBH or gating

- IV contrast: 150 cc at 5 cc/sec requires at least 20 gauge IV; timing of scan after injection depends on motion management technique.
  - DIBH: 45 sec and 1.5 min delay from start of injection. Use a 1.0–1.5 min delay if only one scan is possible (hepatic venous or late portal venous phase).
  - 4D-CT: start both at the same time.
- Isocenter at GTV

CONTOURING:

Target volumes	Definition and description
GTV	All gross disease on imaging, including the primary tumor paying particular attention to extension into/along the vessels (especially HCC), and all suspicious nodes
ITV-optional	If using the ITV approach, use the guidelines for GTV delineation on all phases of the 4D-CT
$CTV_{high\ dose}$	Corresponds to GTV or ITV if used without additional margin
$CTV_{microscopic\ dose}$	GTV + 5 mm Elective nodal irradiation NOT routinely recommended for IHCC or HCC but may be used for hilar cholangiocarcinoma or for N+ tumors at the discretion of the treating physician
$PTV_{high\ dose}$	Uniform expansion $CTV_{high\ dose}$ by 0.5 cm followed by subtraction of any overlapping critical OAR (stomach, small bowel, large bowel) with additional safety margin of 0.5 cm. EXCEPTION: Craniocaudal margin of 1.0 cm for lesions in the liver dome if treating with DIBH and setting up to liver shape
$PTV_{microscopic\ dose}$	PTV margin is based on the motion management technique used (if any) and should be at least 0.5 cm. No subtraction of OARs is used here.
Notable OAR volumes	Applicable for doses ≥60Gy in 25 fractions (or BED equivalent)
Stomach-Proximal Duodenum PRV	Stomach and duodenum segments 1 and 2 + 3–5 mm
Small Bowel PRV	All other small bowel +3–5 mm
Bile Duct PRV	Bile duct from CBD to and including the second-order bile ducts (e.g., right and left hepatic ducts) + 5 mm. Alternative: Can use PV as a surrogate for bile duct location +10 mm

On Treatment Management and Follow-Up Care

COMMON TOXICITIES:

- Nausea/Vomiting: pretreatment anti-emetics, PPI
- Esophagitis: Diet modification→PPI → Carafate→Opiates

- Diarrhea: Low-fat, low-fiber diet modification → Imodium →. More severe diarrhea is unusual and should prompt a workup.

  FOLLOW-UP SCHEDULE:

- 6–8 weeks post RT: Rad Onc Tox Check, CT liver (4 phase), LFTs, AFP (HCC), CA19–9 (IHCC), CEA (colorectal liver metastasis)
- Follow 3 m with CT and blood work

Rectal Cancer

The role of radiotherapy for rectal cancer has continued to evolve beyond the well-established standard of care of preoperative radiotherapy for planned surgical resection. Patients benefit from selection to avoid overtreatment. Patients with low-lying tumors may be managed with a non-operative approach with a preferred sequence of chemoradiation therapy followed by consolidative chemotherapy and close clinical monitoring. Patients with proximal tumors and a low lymph node burden may be able to undergo chemotherapy and surgery and avoid radiotherapy. Finally, patients with high microsatellite instability can be treated with immunotherapy in the upfront setting.

History and Workup

- Distance from anal verge (AV). If <2–3 cm from AV, include prophylactic coverage of the inguinal and external iliac lymph nodes.
- Anterior organ extension (T4 disease): Include prophylactic coverage of external iliac lymph nodes.
- Pelvic side wall or non-TME lymph nodes: Plan for resection? If not, boost.
- Treatment intent:
  - Neoadjuvant with planned surgery
  - Neoadjuvant with hope for non-operative management
- Tumor characteristics
  - MSI: consider immunotherapy as monotherapy

Imaging

- CT C/A/P and rectal MRI for staging

Planning and Treatment Delivery

- If preference for organ-preservation (OP), induction long-course chemoradiation (LCCRT) consolidation FOLFOX/CapeOx is preferred approach a la OPRA
  - OPRA OP rate at 3-yrs
  - Induction LCCRT ➔ consolidative CTX: 53%
  - Induction CTX ➔ consolidative LCCRT: 41%
- Response assessment 8 weeks post-chemotherapy completion with MR rectum, endoscopy, and CT CAP
- Watch and wait (WW) or surgery based on clinical response with decision at discretion of surgeon
- If goal for OP, LCCRT is strongly preferred over short-course RT (SCRT)
  - SCRT is acceptable if the patient is unable to receive concurrent chemotherapy, has distant metastatic disease necessitating continuous multi-agent systemic therapy administration, or other extenuating factors
- If highly symptomatic and/or concern for obstruction: Induction FOLFOX/CapeOX➔consolidation LCCRT based on anecdotal reports that clinical response to CTX is more rapid than RT

DOSES:

- 3DCRT is standard for rectal cancer
- Dose and fractionation
  - Surgery planned

    PTV45: 45 Gy delivered in 25 fractions of 1.8 Gy per day

    PTV50.4: total dose of the PTV50.4 will include the initial 45 Gy followed by a sequential 'cone-down' boost of 5.4 Gy delivered in 3 fractions of 1.8 Gy per day (total dose of 50.4 Gy)

    Daily KV imaging match to bone recommended given setup uncertainty with prone positioning

    Alternatively, SCRT can be offered at 25 Gy in 5 fractions
  - Organ preservation

    PTV45: PTV45 will be 45 Gy delivered in 25 fractions of 1.8 Gy per day

    PTV54: total dose of the PTV54 will include the initial 45 Gy followed by a sequential 'cone-down' boost of 9 Gy delivered in 5 fractions of 1.8 Gy per day (total dose of 54 Gy)

    Daily KV imaging match to bone recommended given setup uncertainty with prone positioning
- IMRT should be considered for the following:
  - Small bowel in pelvis that cannot be spared (Can consider comfortably full bladder)
  - Fixed small bowel
  - Low-lying tumors (<2–3 cm of AV or clearly distal to the dentate line); IMRT indicated to treat the inguinal and external iliac vessels to spare genitalia

  - Lateral pelvic, non-TME, or inguinal lymph nodes that will not be resected should be boosted
- Dose and fractionation
  - Surgery planned

    Simultaneous integrated boost

    PTV45: 45 Gy delivered in 25 fractions of 1.8 Gy per day

    PTV50: 50 Gy delivered in 25 fractions of 2.0 Gy per day

    Optional pelvic sidewall/inguinal/non-TME nodal boost 62.5Gy in 25 fractions (SIB)

    SCRT is an acceptable alternative

    - PTV25: 25 Gy delivered in 5 fractions of 5.0 Gy per day
    - Optional pelvic sidewall/inguinal/non-TME nodal boost 30–40 Gy in 5 fractions
  - Hope for organ preservation

    PTV47: 46.98Gy delivered in 27 fractions of 1.74 Gy per day

    PTV54: 54 Gy delivered in 27 fractions of 2.0 Gy per day

    Optional pelvic sidewall/inguinal/non-TME nodal boost 62.91Gy in 27 fractions (SIB)

    Alternatively, sequential boost

SIMULATION:

- Prone, belly board (alterative prone with Aquaplast mold)
- PO contrast is recommended to aid small bowel contour
- Consider IV contrast for bulky LAD, non-TME LNs
- If small bowel in pelvis, consider comfortably full bladder switching to IMRT
- If IMRT, supine, alpha cradle with recommendation for PO and IV contrast. Vaginal dialators for tumors extending into anal canal.
- BLADDER FILLING: If bladder distension is preferred, coach the patient and use CBCT as needed to optimize volume while providing feedback to the patient. It does not need to be maximally filled or the same shape from day to day.

CONTOURING:

- GTV: Contour the primary GTV and nodal GTV separately
- CTV45 or CTV47: Includes the GTV +1.5 cm margin and also areas at risk for harboring microscopic disease.
  - The CTV45/47 should include the mesorectum (perirectal fat and the presacral space) and internal iliac lymph nodes.
  - If a T4 tumor involves GU/GYN organs, the CTV45 will include the same structures as for a T1–3 tumor but will also include the external iliac lymph nodes
  - If radiographically suspicious common iliac or para-aortic lymph nodes, extend CTV 45 superiorly to the diaphragm

- CTV50 or CTV54 based on treatment intent: Defined as the gross disease (primary and nodal disease) plus a 1.5 cm margin, along with the entire mesorectum (in the region of the tumor and any gross nodes, CT sim slices that include gross disease) modified to remove barriers to anatomical spread such as muscle, bone, and organs.
  - If a low tumor can extend the CTV50/54 superiorly to cover the mesorectum to the sacroiliac notch
- PTV45/47: CTV45 + 0.5 cm symmetric margin
- PTV50/54: CTV50 or CTV 54 + 0.5 cm symmetric margin
- Organs at risk (OARs)
  - Bowel_Sm
  - Bowel_Lg
  - Rectum
  - Bladder
  - External Genitalia
  - Optional:
    Testes
    Ovaries, though required if s/p ovarian transposition
    Anal Canal

Rectal Re-Irradiation

DOSES:

- Preferred BID to 39 Gy, with conedown to 45 Gy.
- Alterative fractionation 30–36 Gy in 1.8 Gy daily fractions.

CONTOURING:

- GTV defined as gross disease on imaging, endoscopy, and clinical exam
- CTV39: defined as the gross disease plus a 1.5 cm margin modified to remove barriers to anatomical spread such as muscle, bone, and organs.
- Elective nodal coverage is dependent on case, prior radiation, duration from prior RT, and anatomy
- PTV39: CTV39 + 0.5 cm
- PTV45: GTV + 0.5 cm

On Treatment Management and Follow-Up Care

COMMON TOXICITIES:

- Dermatitis:
  - Emollients: Consider moisturizer and Desitin/Coloplast prophylactically

  - Silvadene for G2 dermatitis
  - Sitz baths, domeboro soaks, lidocaine, oral opiates, topical morphine sulfate 0.75 g compound QID
  - Consider WOC or dermatology referral if grade 3+ toxicity
    - Per dermatology, avoid medium-to-high-potency steroids for the perineum
- Diarrhea: Low-fat, low-fiber diet modification (BRAT diet)
  - Imodium→Lomotil→Opium→Chemo dose adjustment or discontinuation→RT break
- Neutropenia: Hold RT for ANC <0.5. Resume once >0.5
- Thrombocytopenia: Hold RT for platelets <25
- Radiation Proctitis
  - *Acute Symptoms*: Manage with antidiarrheals, hydration, pain control, topical steroids (proctofoam), PRN
  - *Chronic Symptoms* (>6 months after RT):
    - Sucralfate Enemas (20 mL of a 10% sucralfate suspension in water) BID until remission of symptoms
  - Refractory Symptoms
    - Referral for APC (Argon Plasma Coagulation)
    - Consider Hyberbaric oxygen
    - Discussion with surgery for palliative diversion for severe refractory cases
- Sexual AEs:
  - ED: If patient motivated, consider prophylactic Viagra 20 mg daily. Start 3 days before start, continue for 12–24 months
    - A list of contraindications to PDE5 inhibitors is provided for reference.
      - Nitrates
      - Alpha-blockers
        - Tamsulosin is the best option here, but should be started at the lowest dose
    - This is not an all-encompassing list, and if in doubt best practice would be to liaise with the patient's primary cardiology team
  - All female patients should be referred to sexual medicine regardless of sexual activity
    - All-encompassing service focused on vaginal health, including topical hormonal replacement
  - Anorectal function: Strongly consider referral for pelvic floor PT for all patients, male and female alike
- **Rectal Follow-Up Schedule**
  - Recommend 1 month follow-up to ensure patient recovered from treatment
  - Thereafter, as per MD acknowledging that most patients will be followed by surgery and medical oncology

Anal Cancer

CRT has replaced radical surgical resection as the cornerstone of treatment for anal SCC since the 1970s, and has served as the model for organ preservation approaches. IMRT reduces treatment toxicity and has been accepted as the standard of care technique based on the results of the phase 2 RTOG 0529 trial.

History and Workup

HPV status

Tumor and lymph node size determine dose and fractionation

Imaging

PET/CT and/or CT chest/abdomen/pelvis with IV contrast

MR for T4 disease

Planning and Treatment Delivery

Concurrent chemoradiation therapy with Capecitabine and MMC on Day 1 +/– Day 28.

DOSES:

Primary

TX and T1: 50 Gy/ 25 fx SIB to primary and 43 Gy microscopic

T2: 54Gy /27 SIB and 45 Gy microscopic

T3 58Gy /29 SIB and 47Gy microscopic

T4 58Gy /29 SIB and 47Gy microscopic

Nodes (all with no CTV/5mm PTV within the microscopic dose above):

<2cm 50Gy SIB

2-5 cm 54Gy* SIB

>5cm 58* SIB

*beware of small bowel in boost. If present consider carve out of SIB.

Always treat paraortic nodes if radiographically suspicious with 2 vertebral body margin above.

Use a vaginal dilator for simulation and throughout treatment to spare long term sexual function. It is critical to spare the external gentitalia and introitus as this is what compromises sexual function. The dilator identifes and displaces the avoidance structure. Do not try to spare the vagina, it is surrounded by nodes at risk.

SIMULATION:

- Supine, alpha cradle, frog leg, anal BB
- Vaginal dilator (placed by patient)
- IV contrast, PO contrast optional, IMRT (no full bladder)

CONTOURING:

- Contour normal structures: rectum, anal canal, small bowel, large bowel and external genitalia. Dosimetrists will contour the bladder, cauda, and femoral heads.
- Contour GTV primary and GTV nodes
- Contour CTVmicroscopic_dose
  - Use CTVA, CTVB, and CTVC from the RTOG atlas (can just make as one structure). Also refer to the Australasian Atlas (Ng M et al. Australasian Gastrointestinal Trials Group (AGITG) contouring atlas and planning guidelines for intensity-modulated radiotherapy in anal cancer. Int J Radiat Oncol Biol Phys. 2012 Aug 1;83(5):1455–62).
  - Note caudal extent of elective CTV for inguinal node per RTOG Atlas is 2 cm below the saphenous/femoral vein junction OR bottom of the lesser trochanter (for node-negative patients). For patients with inguinal N+, it needs to be at least 1 cm below the lowest node.
  - CTVC from RTOG atlas is skimpy in the inguinal lymph node basins. Australasian atlas (reference above) is a better atlas to use here.
- Expand each CTV by 5 mm to make each PTV

Anorectal Melanoma

- 25 Gy in 5 Gy per fraction to CTV-A based on NRG contouring atlas
- SIB of 30 Gy/5 fractions with modest GTV to PTV margin
- 2 fractions per week with at least 1 day of rest in between

On Treatment Management and Follow-Up Care

- Dermatitis:
  - Emollients: Consider moisturizer and Desitin/Coloplast prophylactically
  - Silvadene for G2 dermatitis
  - Sitz baths, domeboro soaks, lidocaine, oral opiates, topical morphine sulfate 0.75 g compound QID
  - Consider WOC or dermatology referral if grade 3+ toxicity

    Per dermatology, avoid medium-to-high-potency steroids for the perineum
- Diarrhea: Low fat, low fiber diet modification (BRAT diet)
  - Imodium→Lomotil→Opium→Chemo dose adjustment or discontinuation→RT break
- Neutropenia: Hold RT for ANC <0.5. Resume once >0.5
- Thrombocytopenia: Hold RT for platelets <25
- Radiation Proctitis
  - *Acute Symptoms*: Manage with antidiarrheals, hydration, pain control, topical steroids (proctofoam), PRN
  - *Chronic Symptoms* (>6 months after RT):

Sucralfate Enemas (20 mL of a 10% sucralfate suspension in water) BID until remission of symptoms
- Refractory Symptoms
  Referral for APC (Argon Plasma Coagulation)
  Consider hyberbaric oxygen
  Discussion with surgery for palliative diversion for severe refractory cases
- Sexual AEs:
  - ED: If patient motivated, consider prophylactic Viagra 20 mg daily. Start 3 days before start, continue for 12–24 months
    A list of contraindications to PDE5 inhibitors is provided for reference.
    - Nitrates
    - Alpha-blockers
      - Tamsulosin is the best option here, but should be started at the lowest dose

    This is not an all-encompassing list, and if in doubt, best practice would be to liaise with the patient's primary cardiology team
  - All female patients should be referred to sexual medicine regardless of sexual activity
    All-encompassing service focused on vaginal health, including topical hormonal replacement
  - Anorectal function: Strongly consider referral for pelvic floor PT for all patients, male and female alike
- **Anal Cancer Follow Up Schedule**
  - 4 weeks post CRT: Rad Onc Tox Check
  - 3–4 months post CRT: Surgery with endoscopy and repeat imaging for response evaluation
  - q4 months up to 2 years post CRT: Rad Onc/Surgery alternating for DRE/endoscopy
  - q6 months years 2–4: Rad Onc/Surgery alternating for DRE
  - q12 month up to 3 years: CT C/A/P and Med Onc follow up
  - >4 year post CRT: Colorectal Survivorship

Prostate Cancer

7

Craig E. Grossman, Daniel Gorovets,
and Michael J. Zelefsky

History and Workup

Always consider the patient's overall health and estimated life expectancy, as this may impact whether and how to treat the patient's prostate cancer. Essential components of the history and work-up for prostate cancer include [1]:

- Intact prostate
  1. Clinical symptoms (rare, and when present, usually indicate advanced disease): examples include bone pain, spinal cord compression, hematuria, urinary incontinence, urinary retention, constipation, hematochezia, pelvic pain, weight loss/anorexia, anemia
  2. Labs (within 3 months of treatment)
     1. Total and free prostate specific antigen (PSA) (patient should abstain from ejaculation/trauma to perineum for at least 1 week prior to the blood draw); also obtain a free/total PSA ratio, as lower percentages (<10–15%) are associated with increased risk of cancer. Account for 5-alpha reductase inhibitors, which decrease the PSA value by half. Since prostate size can

C. E. Grossman (✉)
Department of Radiation Oncology, University of South Florida Morsani College of Medicine, Tampa, FL, USA
e-mail: grossmanc@usf.edu

D. Gorovets
Department of Radiation Oncology, Memorial Sloan Kettering Cancer Center, New York, NY, USA
e-mail: gorovetd@mskcc.org

M. J. Zelefsky
Department of Radiation Oncology, New York University Langone Medical Center, New York, NY, USA
e-mail: Michael.zelefsky@nyulangone.org

J. J. Cuaron, L. Z. Braunstein (eds.), *Radiation Oncology Clinical Fundamentals*,
https://doi.org/10.1007/978-3-031-77559-8_7

      cause higher PSA levels, a PSA density (PSA level/prostate size) >=0.15 ng/ml/cc should prompt further workup.
   2. Total Testosterone
   3. Complete blood count (CBC), complete metabolic panel (CMP), hemoglobin A1c (HgA1c), vitamin D, and lipid panel should be obtained, especially if patients are being considered for androgen deprivation therapy
3. Physical examination
   1. DRE to assess prostate size, symmetry, palpable nodules, clinical extracapsular extension (ECE)/seminal vesicle invasion (SVI); rectal wall invasion, rectal tone
   2. Assess for inguinal lymphadenopathy and lower extremity edema
   3. Assess for bone pain
4. Baseline urinary (AUA International Prostate Symptom Score (IPSS)), sexual (International Index of Erectile Function (IIEF)), and bowel function (i.e., hemorrhoids, frequency, typical consistency, presence of irritable bowel syndrome (IBS)/inflammatory bowel disease (IBD) and how well it is controlled); if a patient is due for a colonoscopy, it is highly recommended to have that performed prior to radiotherapy to avoid the need of a colonoscopy within the first year of treatment.
5. Biopsy
   1. Historically, a transrectal ultrasound (TRUS) systematic 12-core prostate biopsy has been performed, but there is increasing use of the transperineal technique due to lower infection rates (although it may require more sedation than a TRUS biopsy)
   2. Ideally, obtain an magnetic resonance (MR)-guided prostate targeted fusion biopsy of any PIRADS 3 or higher prostatic nodules

- Post-prostatectomy
  1. Labs
     1. Total and free PSA
     2. Total Testosterone
     3. CBC, CMP, HgA1c, vitamin D, lipid panel, and thyroid function tests should be obtained especially if patients are being considered for androgen deprivation therapy
  2. Physical examination, including DRE, assessment for inguinal lymphadenopathy and lower extremity edema, and assessment for bone pain
  3. Baseline urinary (IPSS), sexual (IIEF), and bowel function (i.e., hemorrhoids, frequency, typical consistency, presence of IBS/IBD, and how well it is controlled); if a patient is due for a colonoscopy, it is highly recommended to have that performed prior to radiotherapy to avoid the need of a colonoscopy within the first year of treatment

Imaging

Key components of the imaging work-up include:

- Intact prostate
  1. Multiparametric MRI prostate w/o contrast
     1. Ideally, obtained prior to a prostate biopsy in effort to target any dominant intraprostatic lesions (DILs); if performed after a biopsy, wait at least 6–8 weeks to avoid post-biopsy changes that can potentially impact interpretation on MRI
     2. Assess for ECE, SVI, pelvic lymphadenopathy, and suspicious osseous lesions
  2. A bone scan for men with unfavorable intermediate- or high-risk disease; can also consider obtaining an MRI whole body with contrast, as this has greater sensitivity than bone scans [2]
  3. DEXA scan for patients who are planned to undergo androgen deprivation therapy (ADT)
  4. Consider PSMA PET/CT in men with high-risk prostate cancer or when there is suspicion of lymph node or distant metastases; with increased utilization due to greater sensitivity and specificity for metastases, PSMA PET/CT scans will likely replace bone scans over time
- Post-prostatectomy
  1. Multiparametric MRI (mpMRI) prostate without contrast to ensure there is no evidence of cancer within the prostate surgical bed, lymph node metastases, or pelvic bone metastases
  2. Bone scan (usually not sensitive with post-prostatectomy PSAs <0.5 ng/ml)
  3. CT chest/abdomen/pelvis (with or without contrast) *or* MRI whole body (with contrast)
  4. DEXA scan for patients who are planned to undergo ADT
  5. Consider PSMA PET/CT (instead of bone scan and CT chest/abdomen/pelvis) due to its greater sensitivity and specificity of lymph node, osseous, and soft tissue metastases

Definitive Prostate Cancer

- **Low-Risk** (≤cT2a, GS 6, PSA <10 ng/ml)
  - Ideally, these patients should undergo active surveillance as treatment does not improve prostate cancer-specific mortality [3]; however, definitive radiation (LDR monotherapy, prostate stereotactic body radiotherapy (SBRT), or moderate hypofractionation) or surgery is appropriate if:
    1. High-volume disease such as multiple core Gleason 6 disease
    2. Intermediate/high Prolaris or Decipher genomic score
    3. Patient preference to pursue treatment
- **Favorable Intermediate-Risk**
  - Definition
    1. Gleason 3 + 4 (with <50% standard template core involvement of Gleason 3 + 3 and/or 3 + 4) and no other intermediate risk factors; *or*
    2. GS 6 with 1 intermediate risk factor (cT2b-c or PSA 10–20 ng/ml)
  - Treatment options

1. Consider active surveillance if a single core has Gleason 3 + 4 disease with <10% of cancer consisting of Gleason 4
2. LDR monotherapy (acceptable even in the presence of *possible* ECE on mpMRI)
3. Prostate SBRT (in the absence of gross/probable ECE on mpMRI, consider adding 6 months of ADT for (a) intraductal component on pathology, or (b) intermediate Decipher genomic score (> = 0.45))
4. In the presence of gross/probable ECE on mpMRI:
   1. Preferably combination HDR prostate brachytherapy boost with EBRT (prostate SBRT preferred, but a 25-fraction course of intensity modulated radiation therapy (IMRT) to the prostate/SVs can also be delivered, especially among patients with higher IPSS scores); consider adding 6 months of ADT for (a) high volume disease (> = 50% positive cores), (b) intraductal component on pathology, or (c) intermediate Decipher genomic score (> =0.45).
   2. Moderate hypofractionation (prostate/SVs) with 6 months of ADT

- **Unfavorable Intermediate-Risk**
  - Definition

1. GS 4 + 3; *or*
2. GS 3 + 4 with ≥50% standard template core involvement (including GS 6 or 7); *or*
3. ≥2 intermediate-risk factors (cT2b-c, GS 7, PSA 10–20 ng/ml)
   - Treatment options

1. Preferred
   1. Combination HDR prostate brachytherapy boost with EBRT (prostate SBRT preferred, but a 25-fraction course of radiation to the prostate/SVs can also be delivered, especially among patients with higher urinary symptom IPSS scores
   2. For those with gross/probable ECE on mpMRI, intraductal component on pathology, or Decipher genomic score > =0.6, we recommend adding a 6 month course of ADT
2. Alternative options
   1. Prostate SBRT with 6 months of ADT
   2. Moderate hypofractionation (prostate/SVs) with 6 months of ADT
   - N.B. For intermediate risk disease, it is not the practice at MSKCC to electively irradiate the pelvic lymph nodes, especially in the absence of any concerning imaging findings

- **High-Risk**
  - Definition: absence of very high-risk features, and only one of the following high-risk features
    1. GS 4 + 4, 3 + 5, or 4 + 5; *or*
    2. cT3a; *or*
    3. PSA >20 ng/ml
  - Treatment options
    1. Preferably, combination HDR prostate brachytherapy boost with 25-fraction whole pelvic IMRT, with 18 months of ADT

2. Alternatively, moderate hypofractionationed whole pelvic IMRT with 18 months of ADT

- **Very High-Risk**
  - Definition
    1. Primary Gleason pattern 5 or > 4 cores GS 8–10; *or*
    2. cT3b-T4; *or*
    3. ≥2 high-risk features (cT3a; GS 4 + 4, 3 + 5, or 4 + 5; PSA >20 ng/ml)
    4. Although standardly defined as metastatic disease, cN+ disease (in the absence of osseous metastases) is treated analogously to very high-risk disease
  - Treatment options
    1. Recommend combination HDR prostate brachytherapy boost with 25-fraction whole pelvic IMRT, with 18–24 months of ADT
    2. Moderate hypofractionated whole pelvic IMRT with 18–24 months of ADT
    3. In very high-risk disease, consider the addition of an androgen receptor signaling inhibitor (ARSI) such as abiraterone [4] or apalutamide [5]

Post-Prostatectomy Radiation

- Generally, early salvage radiotherapy is preferred as opposed to adjuvant radiation (per RADICALS [6], RAVES [7], GETUG [8] randomized studies)
  - Typically, initiate early salvage therapy when the patient has a post-radical prostatectomy biochemical recurrence (defined by the AUA as a PSA ≥0.2 ng/ml on at least two successive blood draws) and < 0.5 ng/ml (as outcomes significantly decline with higher PSAs [9])
  - Situations to consider *adjuvant* radiation (instead of early salvage radiation) once the patient has had adequate urinary recovery include

    Positive surgical margins

    pT3-4 GS 8-10

    Pathological lymph node metastases

- Specific scenarios
  - Urinary incontinence

    Salvage/adjuvant radiation should preferably be delayed until the patient's urinary continence plateaus (usually takes about 6 months post-prostatectomy)

    - Encourage patients to perform Kegel exercises regularly
    - May need to refer patient for urodynamic studies in the presence of persistent urinary incontinence
    - If the patient requires an artificial sphincter, radiation should not start until at least 3 months after placement of a device; if radiation is initiated first, then a device is placed at least 3 months after completing radiation
  - Radiographically suspicious *prostate bed recurrent/residual disease*: consider pathologic confirmation and fiducial marker placement (for subsequent image-guided boost to the prostate bed gross disease)
  - Radiographically suspicious *lymph node or osseous metastasis*: consider pathologic confirmation

Planning and Treatment Delivery

Definitive Prostate Cancer Treatment

- Radiation treatment regimens
  1. Active surveillance
     1. PSA every 6 months
     2. DREs at follow-ups, especially between scheduled MRIs and biopsies
     3. mpMRI prostate without contrast every 18 months
     4. Prostate biopsy every 3 years; sooner if there is a change in screening mpMRI or PSA
        1. Often, an initial confirmatory biopsy might be performed earlier
        2. For older patients or those with medical co-morbidities, consider increasing the time interval between biopsies to minimize risk of complications
  2. LDR monotherapy
     1. Eligibility
        1. Prostate gland ≤60 cc, to avoid pubic arch interference; in the case of larger glands, consider downsizing with 3 months of ADT
        2. IPSS ≤18
        3. No prior major procedures to the prostate (i.e., cryotherapy, TURP, HIFU)
        4. Prefer LDR brachytherapy over SBRT in patients with IBS/IBD
     2. Dose to Prostate/SVs: 144 Gy (I-125) or 125 Gy (Pd-103)
     3. Consider rectal spacer implants to reduce exposure of the rectum to higher radiation dose levels
  3. SBRT prostate (with fiducial markers and rectal spacer placed prior to simulation)
     - Dose to Prostate/SVs: 40 Gy (8 Gy × 5 fx, every other day).
     - In patients who desire prostate SBRT but cannot undergo rectal pacer implantation (i.e., presence of posterior ECE, contraindications to sedation/anesthesia, not technically feasible, other logistics), consider *proton* SBRT, MR-guided SBRT, or decreasing the SBRT dose to 35–37.5 Gy if normal rectal dose constraints cannot be achieved
  4. HDR prostate brachytherapy followed by EBRT (SBRT or conventionally fractionated IMRT)
     1. Eligibility
        1. Prostate gland ≤60 cc; in the case of larger glands, consider downsizing with 3 months of ADT
        2. IPSS ≤20
        3. No prior major procedures to the prostate (i.e., cryotherapy, TURP, HIFU)
     2. Rectal spacer implant (assuming no evidence of gross/suspicious posterior ECE on mpMRI) and fiducial markers are placed immediately after prostate brachytherapy

3. Dose
    1. HDR prostate brachytherapy: 15 Gy × 1
    2. EBRT portion
        1. SBRT (Prostate/SVs): 25 Gy (5 Gy × 5 fx, qd)
        2. Conventional IMRT (Prostate/SVs): 45 Gy (1.8 Gy × 25 fx, qd)
        3. Conventional IMRT (Whole Pelvis)
            1. Prostate/SVs & Elective Pelvic LNs: 45 Gy (1.8 Gy × 25 fx, qd)
            2. In the presence of suspicious LN metastases, treat with SIB: 56.25 Gy (2.25 Gy × 25 fx, qd)

5. Moderate hypofractionation (with fiducial markers placed prior to simulation)
    1. Prostate/SVs: 70.2 Gy (2.7 Gy × 26 fx, qd)
    2. Pelvic LNs: 46.8 Gy (1.8 Gy × 26 fx, qd)
    3. In the presence of suspicious LN metastases, treat with SIB: 57.2 Gy (2.2 Gy × 26 fx, qd)

- ADT regimens
    - Neoadjuvant/concurrent/adjuvant ADT, beginning approximately 2–3 months prior to delivery of radiation
        1. Typically, we administer 3-month leuprolide injections (22.5 mg IM), with the addition of bicalutamide 50 mg q day if PSA level does not nadir to undetectable levels within 3 months of initiating leuprolide; bicalutamide can be discontinued when RT is completed
        2. Alternative hormonal agents (i.e., degarelix or relugolix) can be used in cases of concern for compliance due to toxicities, cardiovascular risk, and/or testosterone recovery
    - Consider 18–24 months ARSIs (i.e., abiraterone or apalutamide) in patients <75 yo without significant comorbidities with Gleason 8–10, PSA > 40 ng/ml, and rT3a/rT3b

- Simulation
    - *MRCAT simulation* is typically performed at MSK. If patient cannot undergo an MRCAT simulation (i.e., bilateral hip replacements, gunshot wounds, wide separation, multiple stents, AICD/PPM, anxiety), a CT simulation with Foley catheter (to visualize the urethra) is performed
        1. Simulation *and* treatments should be scheduled to occur after a patient typically has a bowel movement to minimize rectal volume
        2. Patient should have a *comfortably* full bladder for simulation and treatments, which is generally achieved by drinking 1 cup (8 oz) of water 45 minutes prior to simulation and treatments, assuming the patient is well-hydrated
        3. Encourage patients to minimize consumption of gas-producing foods/drinks a few days prior to simulation and throughout treatment in an attempt to minimize rectal volume
    - Positioning: Supine, arms on chest, aquaplast immobilization
    - Isocenter: prostate (when only prostate/SVs are being treated), top of femoral heads (when elective pelvic lymph nodes are being treated).

- Contouring
  - Normal structures
    1. Small bowel and large bowel, at least 2 cm superior and inferior from the treatment field
    2. Rectum
    3. Bladder
    4. Bladder trigone (for SBRT cases only)
    5. Penile bulb
    6. Femoral heads
    7. Cauda
    8. Rectal spacer (when present)
    9. Fiducial markers (when present)
  - Target volumes
    1. CTV_Prostate: prostate (include median lobe) and *proximal half* of seminal vesicles (*however, if there is significant disease in the base, then include entire SVs in the CTV*)
       1. Ensure CTV encompasses the ECE
       2. Contour the DIL(s), even though it may not be targeted specifically, to ensure it is receiving sufficient prescription dose
    2. PTV_Prostate = CTV + 0.3 cm circumferentially
    3. Elective Pelvic LNs (high-risk disease)
       1. CTV_LN: 0.5 cm margin around vessels, starting at the common iliac bifurcation (which is approximately the top of L4/5), according to the NRG regional pelvic nodal atlas [10]
          1. *In the presence of suspicious LN metastases in the pelvic region* (below common iliacs, i.e., the aortic bifurcation), the elective LN field should be extended above the bifurcation (~top of L3)
          2. *In the presence of suspicious LN metastases in the common iliac/para-aortic region*, the elective LN field should be extended no higher than the level of the renal hilum (i.e., to approximately L1/L2) to electively cover the para-aortic LNs; consider covering only the lower para-aortic LNs for suspicious common iliac lymph node involvement
          3. *In the presence of suspicious LN metastases in the mesorectum*, the elective LN field should include the entire mesorectum (following rectal cancer contouring guidelines)
             1. Do not carve out the rectum
             2. Superior border: rectosigmoid flexure; inferior border: anorectal junction
  - 2. PTV_LN: CTV_LN + 0.5 cm

    4. Simultaneous boost for suspicious LN metastases
       1. PTV_LN_Boost: GTV_LN_Boost + 0.5 cm
    - Organ motion monitoring
      - Prostate SBRT

1. Daily kV (matched to fiducial markers) and CBCTs (to confirm target coverage and rectal/bladder volumes)
2. Daily intrafractional monitoring [11]
   - Moderate Hypofractionation IMRT
1. Daily kV (matched to fiducial markers)
2. At least twice/week CBCTs (to confirm target coverage and rectal/bladder volumes)
3. Daily intrafractional monitoring [11]
   - Post-brachytherapy 25 fraction IMRT
1. Daily kV (matched to fiducial markers)
2. At least twice/week CBCTs (to confirm target coverage and rectal/bladder volumes)
3. Daily intrafractional monitoring [11]

Post-Prostatectomy Cancer Treatment

- Treatment regimen
  - 6 months of neoadjuvant/concurrent/adjuvant ADT
    1. Begin approximately 2 months prior to delivery of radiation
    2. Typically, we administer 3-month leuprolide injections (22.5 mg IM), with the addition of bicalutamide 50 mg q day if PSA level does not nadir to undetectable levels within 3 months of initiating leuprolide; bicalutamide can be discontinued when RT is completed
    3. Alternative hormonal agents (i.e., degarelix or relugolix) can be used in cases of concern for compliance due to toxicities, cardiovascular risk, and/or testosterone recovery
  - In patients with suspicious or pathologically-confirmed LN metastases, consider 18–24 months ADT with the addition of an ARSI
  - Deliver salvage radiation to both the prostate bed and elective pelvic lymph nodes with ADT, based on the results of NRG/RTOG 0534 [12]
    1. In patients with IBS/IBD, low clinical suspicion of pelvic LN microscopic disease, or those who had an extensive negative lymph node dissection, consider omitting pelvic LN irradiation
    2. Boost suspicious prostate bed recurrent/residual disease (if fiducial markers have been placed prior to simulation)
  - Consider salvage radiation *without ADT* in the following situations: multiple comorbidities including cardiac and/or neurologic/psychiatric, advanced age (>80 yo), patient refusal
  - Conventional IMRT dose regimen (note, we are starting to adopt moderate hypofractionated regimens, given the results of such studies as GU003 [13]
    1. Prostatectomy bed
       1. 66.6 Gy (1.8 Gy × 37 fx, qd): *when delivered with ADT* in the setting of a negative PSMA PET scan
       2. 72 Gy (1.8 Gy × 40 fx, qd)

        1. If there is suspicion of prostate bed recurrent/residual disease (either via imaging or biopsy) or post-prostatectomy positive/close surgical margin.
        2. In the absence of ADT.
    2. Elective Pelvic LNs: 45 Gy (1.8 Gy × 25 fx, qd).
    3. Suspicious LN metastases: 56.25 Gy (2.25 Gy × 25 fx, qd).
    4. Suspicious prostate bed recurrent/residual disease: 78 Gy (1.8 Gy × 40 fx, qd → 2 Gy × 3 fx, qd).

- Simulation
  - MRCAT or CT simulation
    1. Simulation *and* treatments should be scheduled to occur after a patient typically has a bowel movement to minimize rectal volume
    2. Patient should have a *comfortably* full bladder for simulation and treatments, which is generally achieved by drinking 1 cup (8 oz) of water 45 minutes prior to simulation and treatments, assuming the patient is well-hydrated
    3. Encourage patients to minimize consumption of gas-producing foods/drinks a few days prior to simulation and throughout treatment in an attempt to minimize rectal volume
  - Positioning: Supine, arms on chest, aquaplast immobilization
  - Isocenter
    1. Prostatectomy bed alone: AP: center on pubic symphysis; lateral: anterior to rectum
    2. When elective pelvic lymph nodes are being treated: top of femoral heads
- Contouring
  - Normal structures
    1. Small bowel and large bowel, at least 2 cm superior and inferior of the treatment field
    2. Rectum
    3. Bladder
    4. Penile bulb
    5. Femoral heads
    6. Cauda
    7. Fiducial markers (when present)
  - Target volumes
    1. Prostatectomy bed
        1. CTV_Prostate_Bed
        1. *Caudally, begin just above GUD*
        2. *Identify vesicourethral anastomosis (VUA) as a slice below last with urine and begin contouring 8–12 mm below*
        3. *At the superior border of pubic symphysis, pull back the anterior border gradually over 3–4 slices to the 3-mm margin allowed on the bladder, forming the classic "dumbbell" shape*
        4. *Cranial border should extend approximately 2 cm above the pubic symphysis, but it is not necessary to encompass all hemostatic clips*

5. *Laterally bound by obturator internus muscle*
2. PTV_Prostate_Bed = CTV + [0.5 cm (lateral, posterior), 0.6 cm (anterior), 0.2 cm (superior, inferior)]
2. Elective Pelvic LNs
   1. CTV_LN: 0.5 cm margin around vessels, starting at the common iliac bifurcation (which is approximately the top of L4/5), according to the NRG regional pelvic nodal atlas [10]
      1. *In the presence of suspicious LN metastases in the pelvic region* (below common iliacs, i.e., the aortic bifurcation), the elective LN field should be extended above the bifurcation (~top of L3)
      2. *In the presence of suspicious LN metastases in the common iliac/para-aortic region* elective LN field should be extended no higher than the level of the renal hilum (i.e., to approximately L1/L2) to electively cover the para-aortic LNs; consider covering only the lower para-aortic LNs for suspicious common iliac lymph node involvement
      3. *In the presence of suspicious LN metastases in the mesorectum*, the elective LN field should include the entire mesorectum (following rectal cancer contouring guidelines)
         1. Do not carve out the rectum
         2. Superior border: rectosigmoid flexure; inferior border: anorectal junction
   - 2. PTV_LN: CTV_LN + 0.5 cm
3. Simultaneous boost for suspicious LN metastases
   1. PTV_LN_Boost: GTV_LN_Boost + 0.5 cm
4. Suspicious prostate bed recurrent/residual disease
   1. PTV_Prostate_Bed_Boost: GTV_Prostate_Bed_Boost + 0.5 cm

- Organ Motion monitoring
  - Daily kV (matched to bone) and twice-weekly CBCTs (to confirm target coverage and rectal/bladder volumes)
  - Daily CBCTs during boost to suspicious prostate bed recurrent/residual disease (to confirm target coverage, ideally matched to fiducials)

On Treatment Management and Follow-Up Care

Common acute toxicities

- Irritative urinary symptoms/bladder spasm/dysuria:
  1. Ibuprofen 400 mg TID (decrease dose or avoid if poor renal function or on anticoagulants)
  2. Phenazopyridine 200 mg TID (reduce dose if poor renal function)
  3. Steroids
  4. Solifenacin or oxybutynin
  5. Tamsulosin

- UTI: order urine culture and treat according to antibiotic sensitivity
- Diarrhea: Loperamide (start with 1/2 tablet daily and can increase dosage, especially on days with loose bowel movements/diarrhea)
- Bowel spasms/tenesmus: Hyoscyamine 0.125 mg QID
- Erectile dysfunction
  1. For patients who are sexually active and/or interested in preserving sexual function: Prescribe sildenafil 20–25 mg daily (start at least 3 days prior to ADT or EBRT, whichever is first) and continue up to 2 years after completing *all* treatments (including ADT); consider also adding 100 mg every fourth day, and encourage penile rehabilitation (attempt to have an erection every few days).
- ADT-specific toxicities: hot flashes (consider SSRIs, fezolinetant, gabapentin, acupuncture), changes in body composition and metabolism (recommend exercise, healthy eating, adjustment of diabetic medications), fatigue, depression/anxiety (refer to social work/therapist; consider anti-depressant), potential cardiovascular effects (if present, refer to cardiology to ensure ADT administration is relatively "safe"), skin rash (with apalutamide, treat with topical steroids), electrolyte abnormalities.

Common late toxicities

- Obstructive urinary symptoms
  1. Start tamsulosin 0.4 mg qhs (or other α-blockers) in naïve patients
  2. Increase the tamsulosin dose to 0.4 mg BID (or 0.8 mg QHS) for patients already on tamsulosin
- Irritative urinary symptoms: Perform a bladder scan.
  1. If PVR <150 cc, prescribe solifenacin or oxybutynin
  2. If PVR >150 cc and have maximized medical therapy (α-blockers and at least 3 months of 5α-reductase inhibitors such as finasteride), refer to a urology for urodynamic studies
- Urinary incontinence: refer to urologist for consideration of artificial sphincter placement
- Rectal: refer to gastroenterology if fail conservative and medical management.
  1. Altered bowel movements
  2. Intermittent rectal bleeding
- Sexual
  1. Erectile dysfunction: if no improvement with daily sildenafil, refer to a sexual health physician for management
  2. Decreased ejaculate volume

Follow-up

- Years 1–2 (evaluation at 3, 6, 12, 18, and 24 months post-radiation treatment): PSA and testosterone level
- At 2-year follow-up, consider a surveillance prostate biopsy for confirmation of local control status in those patients treated with SBRT or combined brachytherapy/SBRT [14]

- After 2 years, PSA and testosterone levels should be obtained annually
- Patients should avoid undergoing a coloscopy within the first year of radiation treatment due to the increased risk of procedure-related rectal/bowel complications

References

1. Siegel RL, Miller KD, Fuchs HE, Jemal A. Cancer statistics, 2022. CA Cancer J Clin. 2022;72(1):7–33.
2. Oprea-Lager DE, Cysouw MCF, Boellaard R, Deroose CM, de Geus-Oei LF, Lopci E, Bidaut L, Herrmann K, Fournier LS, Bäuerle T, deSouza NM, Lecouvet FE. Bone Metastases Are Measurable: The Role of Whole-Body MRI and Positron Emission Tomography. Front Oncol. 2021;11:772530. https://doi.org/10.3389/fonc.2021.772530. PMID: 34869009; PMCID: PMC8640187.
3. Hamdy FC, Donovan JL, Lane JA, Metcalfe C, Davis M, Turner EL, et al. Fifteen-year outcomes after monitoring, surgery, or radiotherapy for prostate cancer. N Engl J Med. 2023;388(17):1547–58.
4. James ND, de Bono JS, Spears MR, Clarke NW, Mason MD, Dearnaley DP, et al. Abiraterone for prostate cancer not previously treated with hormone therapy. N Engl J Med. 2017;377(4):338–51.
5. Chi KN, Agarwal N, Bjartell A, et al. Apalutamide for metastatic, castration-sensitive prostate cancer. N Engl J Med 2019;381:13-24. Available at: https://www.ncbi.nlm.nih.gov/pubmed/31150574.
6. Parker CC, Clarke NW, Cook AD, Kynaston HG, Petersen PM, Catton C, et al. Timing of radiotherapy after radical prostatectomy (RADICALS-RT): a randomised, controlled phase 3 trial. Lancet. 2020;396(10260):1413–21.
7. Kneebone A, Fraser-Browne C, Duchesne GM, Fisher R, Frydenberg M, Herschtal A, et al. Adjuvant radiotherapy versus early salvage radiotherapy following radical prostatectomy (TROG 08.03/ANZUP RAVES): a randomised, controlled, phase 3, non-inferiority trial. Lancet Oncol. 2020;21(10):1331–40.
8. Sargos P, Chabaud S, Latorzeff I, Magne N, Benyoucef A, Supiot S, et al. Adjuvant radiotherapy versus early salvage radiotherapy plus short-term androgen deprivation therapy in men with localised prostate cancer after radical prostatectomy (GETUG-AFU 17): a randomised, phase 3 trial. Lancet Oncol. 2020;21(10):1341–52.
9. Tendulkar RD, Agrawal S, Gao T, Efstathiou JA, Pisansky TM, Michalski JM, et al. Contemporary update of a multi-institutional predictive nomogram for salvage radiotherapy after radical prostatectomy. J Clin Oncol. 2016;34(30):3648–54.
10. Hall WA, Paulson E, Davis BJ, Spratt DE, Morgan TM, Dearnaley D, et al. NRG oncology updated international consensus atlas on pelvic lymph node volumes for intact and postoperative prostate cancer. Int J Radiat Oncol Biol Phys. 2021;109(1):174–85.
11. Gorovets D, Burleson S, Jacobs L, Ravindranath B, Tierney K, Kollmeier M, et al. Prostate SBRT with intrafraction motion management using a novel linear accelerator-based MV-kV imaging method. Pract Radiat Oncol. 2020;10(5):e388–e96.
12. Pollack A, Karrison TG, Balogh AG, Gomella LG, Low DA, Bruner DW, et al. The addition of androgen deprivation therapy and pelvic lymph node treatment to prostate bed salvage radiotherapy (NRG Oncology/RTOG 0534 SPPORT): an international, multicentre, randomised phase 3 trial. Lancet. 2022;399(10338):1886–901.
13. Buyyounouski MK, Pugh SL, Chen RC, et al. Noninferiority of Hypofractionated vs Conventional Postprostatectomy Radiotherapy for Genitourinary and Gastrointestinal Symptoms: The NRG-GU003 Phase 3 Randomized Clinical Trial. JAMA Oncol. 2024;10(5):584–591. https://doi.org/10.1001/jamaoncol.2023.729.
14. Gorovets D, Wibmer AG, Moore A, Lobaugh S, Zhang Z, Kollmeier M, et al. Local failure after prostate SBRT predominantly occurs in the PI-RADS 4 or 5 dominant intraprostatic lesion. Eur Urol Oncol. 2022;6:275.

Bladder Cancer

8

Craig E. Grossman

Abbreviations

CBC	Complete blood count
CMP	Complete metabolic panel
DRE	Digital rectal exam
eGFR	Estimated glomerular filtration rate
OR	Operating room
TMT	Trimodality definitive therapy
TURBT	Transurethral resection of bladder tumor
UTIs	Urinary tract infections

History and Workup

Essential components of the history and work-up for bladder cancer include:

- Clinical symptoms: Gross or microscopic painless hematuria, irritative or obstructive voiding symptoms; pain (i.e., flank, suprapubic, rectal/perineal, bone), fatigue, weight loss, and/or anorexia may suggest locally advanced or metastatic disease
- Risk factor assessment: smoking history, occupational exposures (aromatic amines, dyes, leather industry, paints); risk factors for squamous cell histology include Schistosoma haematobium infection (prevalent in developing countries) and prolonged bladder inflammation (usually from long-term indwelling Foley catheter or chronic UTIs)

C. E. Grossman (✉)
Department of Radiation Oncology, University of South Florida Morsani College of Medicine, Tampa, FL, USA
e-mail: grossmanc@usf.edu

J. J. Cuaron, L. Z. Braunstein (eds.), *Radiation Oncology Clinical Fundamentals*, https://doi.org/10.1007/978-3-031-77559-8_8

- Physical examination: DRE to assess prostate/rectal invasion; bimanual exam in women to assess vaginal/uterine involvement; pelvic/inguinal lymph node evaluation
- Labs: CBC and CMP, with attention to eGFR for cisplatin eligibility and/or need for stent placement
- Urinalysis and urine cytology
- Cystoscopy with maximal TURBT of all visible tumors (preferred) or biopsy, with placement of fiducial markers to demarcate the involved area.
  - Usually, an office cystoscopy with biopsy is initially performed to establish a diagnosis, followed by a more extensive cystoscopy in the OR with general anesthesia to map out the extent of the tumor with a maximal TURBT
- Assessment of candidacy for TMT: absence of moderate/severe hydronephrosis, without concurrent extensive or multifocal carcinoma in situ (CIS), <6 cm unifocal tumor that can be maximally debulked, no prior pelvic radiation, and adequate pre-treatment bladder function and capacity

Imaging

Key components of the imaging work-up include:

- CT of the abdomen and pelvis (CT urogram) with and without contrast, with excretory imaging; can also consider MR abdomen/pelvis as an alternative (especially in patients with poor renal function/iodine allergy)
- FDG PET/CT is now more commonly being used to assess for metastatic disease. Otherwise, CT chest is required with full-body bone imaging

Planning and Treatment Delivery

- A bladder-sparing approach of definitive chemoradiation should commence as soon as possible following maximal TURBT (ideally within 4 weeks, but not more than 8 weeks).
- Although concurrent cisplatin (+/− 5-FU) or 5-FU/Mitomycin C are most commonly used as radiosensitizers for bladder cancer, we typically favor the use of low-dose biweekly gemcitabine (25 mg/m^2) due to less toxicity with comparable disease control rates [1].
- Radiation treatment volumes, techniques, and doses vary across clinical trials and institutions. IMRT is preferred over 3D-CRT [2] to spare adjacent bowel, rectum, femurs, and spinal cord/cauda.

  DOSES:

- Based on a meta-analysis of two randomized controlled trials (BC2001 [3] and BCON [4]) that concluded the hypofractionated schedule of 55 Gy in 20 fractions was non-inferior to 64 Gy in 32 fractions in regard to both locoregional control and late bladder and rectal toxicity [5], we favor use of the 55 Gy regimen, especially in cases of clinically node-negative disease, patients with multiple comorbidities/older age/poor performance status, and/or multifocal disease

- Whole bladder: 55 Gy in 20 fractions (2.75 Gy/fx)
- Whole pelvis and bladder tumor/tumor bed boost or whole bladder: 45 Gy in 25 fractions (1.8 Gy/fx) with a bladder tumor/tumor bed boost or whole bladder to 66.6 Gy (21.6 Gy boost delivered over 12 fractions)

  In the presence of clinically node-positive disease, consider a SIB of 56.25 Gy in 25 fractions (2.25 Gy/fx) for any suspicious LN metastases within the elective nodal field

SIMULATION:

- Supine, arms on chest, aquaplast immobilization
- Consider oral contrast (about 2 hours prior to simulation) and rectal contrast for delineation of the large bowel and rectum, respectively
- Encourage patients to minimize consumption of gas-producing foods/drinks a few days prior to simulation and throughout treatment in an attempt to minimize rectal volume
- For whole bladder only treatment, patients should empty their bladder immediately prior to simulation
- For whole pelvis with bladder tumor/tumor bed boost, patient should be simulated first with a full bladder and then with an empty bladder
- Isocenter: center of bladder

CONTOURING:

- Contour normal structures
  - Small bowel and large bowel, at least 2 cm superior and inferior of the treatment field
  - Rectum
  - Femoral heads
  - Cauda
  - Fiducial markers (when present)
- For whole bladder only treatment
  - CTV_Bladder: entire bladder; CTV_Prostate to cover the prostatic urethra: entire prostate (no seminal vesicles unless they are involved)
  - PTV_Bladder = CTV_Bladder +1.5 cm, CTV_Prostate +0.5 cm
- For whole pelvis and bladder tumor/tumor bed boost treatment
  - CTV_Pelvis (contoured on the empty bladder scan): entire bladder (CTV_Bladder), entire prostate without seminal vesicles unless involved (CTV_Prostate), CTV_Nodes (0.5 cm margin around vessels, according to the NRG reginal pelvic nodal atlas [6])

  - CTV_Bladder Tumor Boost (contoured on the full bladder scan): bladder wall encompassing the fiducial markers delineating the tumor bed, and when available, the bladder map from TURBT; can also fuse the pre-TURBT scan to the simulation scan as a guide for tumor bed delineation
  - PTV_Pelvis (contoured on the empty bladder scan) = CTV_Bladder +1.5 cm, CTV_Prostate +0.5 cm, CTV_Nodes +0.5 cm
  - PTV_Bladder Tumor Boost (contoured on the full bladder scan) = CTV_Bladder Tumor Boost +0.5–1 cm
  - PTV_Node_Boost: radiographic suspicious nodal metastases +0.5 cm

BLADDER-SPARING TREATMENT:

- Whole bladder only: treat with empty bladder
- Whole pelvis and bladder tumor/tumor bed boost
  - Bladder should be empty for treatment of the whole pelvis portion of the plan; bladder should be full during the tumor/tumor bed boost portion of treatment
  - Consider giving the boost upfront (before treating the whole pelvis), as patients may otherwise have difficulty maintaining a full bladder for the boost portion if administered toward the end of treatment
- OBI
  - For whole bladder treatment or the whole pelvis portion of treatment: daily kVs matched to bone, at least twice/week CBCTs to assess bladder fill
  - For bladder tumor/tumor bed boost portion of treatment: daily CBCTs matched to fiducials; match to bladder if there are no fiducials.

On Treatment Management and Follow-Up Care

Common acute toxicities

- Irritative urinary symptoms/bladder spasm/dysuria: Ibuprofen 400 mg TID (decrease dose or avoid if poor renal function or on anticoagulants) → Phenazopyridine 200 mg TID (reduce dose if poor renal function) → Steroids, Solifenacin or Oxybutynin, Tamsulosin
- UTI: order urine culture and treat according to antibiotic sensitivity
- Diarrhea: Loperamide (start with 1/2 tablet daily and can increase dosage, especially on days with loose bowel movements/diarrhea)
- Bowel spasms/tenesmus: Hyoscyamine 0.125 mg QID
- Cytopenia: Medical oncologist to manage

Follow up

- Reassess tumor status 2–3 months after completing treatment with imaging (ideally MRI abdomen/pelvis; otherwise, CT urogram), cystoscopy, and labs (CBC, CMP, U/A, and cytology)

- CBC, CMP, and urine cytology every 3-6 months for at least the first two years
- MRI (preferred) or CT abdomen/pelvis, urine cytology, and cystoscopy at 3–6-month intervals for 2 years; then every 6–12 months for up to 5 years
- For patients who do not achieve a complete response or ultimately recur, salvage cystectomy versus systemic therapy should be considered
- FDG PET/CT scan in patients with suspected metastatic disease

References

1. Oh KS, Soto DE, Smith DC, Montie JE, Lee CT, Sandler HM. Combined-modality therapy with gemcitabine and radiation therapy as a bladder preservation strategy: long-term results of a phase I trial. Int J Radiat Oncol Biol Phys. 2009;74(2):511–7.
2. Sherry AD, Stewart A, Luo G, Kirschner AN. Intensity-Modulated Radiotherapy is Superior to Three-Dimensional Conformal Radiotherapy in the Trimodality Management of Muscle-Invasive Bladder Cancer with Daily Cone Beam Computed Tomography Optimization. J Radiat Oncol. 2019 Dec;8(4):395–403. https://doi.org/10.1007/s13566-019-00411-0. Epub 2019 Dec 18. PMID: 33343830; PMCID: PMC7747671.
3. James ND, Hussain SA, Hall E, Jenkins P, Tremlett J, Rawlings C, et al. Radiotherapy with or without chemotherapy in muscle-invasive bladder cancer. N Engl J Med. 2012;366(16):1477–88.
4. Hoskin PJ, Rojas AM, Bentzen SM, Saunders MI. Radiotherapy with concurrent carbogen and nicotinamide in bladder carcinoma. J Clin Oncol. 2010;28(33):4912–8.
5. Choudhury A, Porta N, Hall E, Song YP, Owen R, MacKay R, et al. Hypofractionated radiotherapy in locally advanced bladder cancer: an individual patient data meta-analysis of the BC2001 and BCON trials. Lancet Oncol. 2021;22(2):246–55.
6. Hall WA, Paulson E, Davis BJ, Spratt DE, Morgan TM, Dearnaley D, et al. NRG oncology updated international consensus atlas on pelvic lymph node volumes for intact and postoperative prostate cancer. Int J Radiat Oncol Biol Phys. 2021;109(1):174–85.

9 Gynecological Cancers

Diana Roth O'Brien, Fumiko Chino, Marisa Kollmeier, and Kaled Alektiar

Endometrial Cancer

Clinical history and Diagnostic Evaluation:

- Abnormal vaginal bleeding /discharge: (quality/timing/duration/extent, last gyn/PAP exam)
- Abdominopelvic symptoms: pain/discomfort, bloating
- Full GYN history: last GYN exam/PAP, parity, history of hormone replacement therapy/tamoxifen)
- Imaging:
  - Transvaginal US: thickened endometrium (>5 mm)
  - CT CAP: performed preoperatively for confirmed endometrial cancer on endometrial biopsy (may be omitted for low-grade disease in the absence of symptoms of distant disease and/or prolonged (>6 m) symptoms)
  - MRI of abdomen/pelvis + CT chest: for suspected high-grade disease may be appropriate
- Surgery: total hysterectomy, bilateral salphingo-oophorectomy and sentinel lymph node sampling or pelvic/para-aortic lymph node dissection
  - Pathology assessment by GYN pathologist preferred
- Medical oncologist consultation
- Genetic risk assessment: screening for Lynch syndrome (MLH1, MSH2, MSH6, PMS2), POLE testing, p53

D. R. O'Brien (✉) · M. Kollmeier · K. Alektiar
Department of Radiation Oncology, Memorial Sloan Kettering Cancer Center, New York, NY, USA
e-mail: rothensd@mskcc.org; kollmeiM@mskcc.org; alektiak@mskcc.org

F. Chino
Department of Radiation Oncology, MD Anderson Cancer Center, Houston, TX, USA
e-mail: fchino@mdanderson.org

J. J. Cuaron, L. Z. Braunstein (eds.), *Radiation Oncology Clinical Fundamentals*,
https://doi.org/10.1007/978-3-031-77559-8_9

Adjuvant Therapy

- Stage I-II (per FIGO 2009 [1])
  - IA, no myometrial invasion, Grade 1/2: observe
  - IA, no myometrial invasion, Grade 3: IVRT (in certain settings observation may also be appropriate, e.g., high risk of toxicity)
  - IA, <50% myometrial invasion, Grade 1/2: observe (if age ≥ 60 or lymphovascular invasion present, IVRT preferred)
  - IA, <50% myometrial invasion, Grade 3: IVRT
  - IB (≥50% myometrial invasion), Grade 1: IVRT
  - IB (≥50% myometrial invasion), Grade 3: pelvic EBRT
  - II, Grades 1–3: pelvic EBRT (IVRT may be reasonable if minimal cervical invasion and/or radical hysterectomy is performed)
  - I-II, serous, clear cell, carcinosarcoma IVRT (with *chemotherapy): observe in settings of no residual tumor in hysterectomy, negative washings
  - +vaginal margins: pelvic EBRT + IVRT boost
  - *if giving pelvic RT, concurrent cisplatin 40 mg/m2 IV
  - *chemotherapy = paclitaxel + carboplatin + 6 cycles
- Stage III-IVa
  - IIIA-IVRT (with *chemotherapy)
    EBRT may be appropriate for patients with contraindications to *chemotherapy)
  - IIIB-EBRT (with *chemotherapy)
  - IIIC1/2-EBRT (with *chemotherapy)
    +measurable residual disease: consider systemic therapy (chemotherapy + immunotherapy for patients who meet eligibility criteria for NRG GY018 [2] or RUBY [3] trials)
    Serous/carcinosarcoma/dedifferentiated (IVRT with chemotherapy)
  - IVa-EBRT (with chemotherapy)
  - *chemotherapy = paclitaxel + carboplatin + 6 cycles
  - *addition of pembrolizumab or dostarlimab (per NRG GY018 [2] and RUBY [3] eligible pts)
  - *HER2/neu positive serous carcinoma: consider addition of trastuzumab

Medically Inoperable [4]

- No myometrial involvement on pretreatment MRI: intracavitary brachytherapy alone (Y applicator)
- +Myometrial involvement or high risk: EBRT + Intracavitary brachytherapy (Y applicator)
- If poor candidate for anesthesia, can consider levonorgestrel-releasing intrauterine device if feasible as alternative to RT (higher endometrial drug concentrations compared with oral therapy with higher response rate and lower toxicity)

Recurrent Disease

- EBRT + IVRT (tumor thickness ≤ 0.5 cm)
- EBRT + Interstitial brachytherapy (tumor thickness > 0.5 cm)

- Techniques:
  - IVRT [5, 6]

    Confirm healed vaginal cuff prior to IVRT (~6–8wks post-op)
    Use maximal cylinder diameter and depth as tolerated
    IVRT delivered weekly
    If IVRT with chemotherapy, IVRT interdigitated between cycles
    Measure vaginal cuff length
    - Treatment length = proximal 2/3 (5–7 cm)
    - Treatment depth = 0.5 cm

    Prescription.
    - ≥3 cm cylinder diameter:700 cGy × 3
    - <3 cm cylinder diameter: 600 cGy × 3
    - In combination with IMRT: 500 cGy × 3

    Treatment verification
    - Dummy wire with AP/lateral films: check consistent treatment depth/cylinder diameter with each fraction

    Medically inoperable: Y applicator with CT/MR plan. Treatment delivered in 3–4 fractions with 1–2 applicator insertions. EQD2 to gross tumor 80–90Gy [4]
    Recurrent disease: multichannel intravaginal cylinder with customized CT/MR plan. Treatment delivered 2–3x/week. For tumors >5 mm thick, use interstitial brachytherapy. Target PTV EQD2 70–75Gy
  - EBRT [7]

    Confirm healed vaginal cuff prior to EBRT (~6 to 8 weeks post-op).
    Supine versus prone position: in general, supine is preferred due to patient comfort; however, small bowel anatomy may be favorable in prone position
    Immobilization: generally used for all. Arms above head when para-aortic nodal regions are included to avoid beam penetration through arms
    Bladder: no filling/emptying instruction
    Contrast
    - Vaginal contrast: given for all. Useful to delineate the superior extent of the vagina cuff. Take care not to overinflate the cuff. BB or wire at introitus to guide inferior extent of PTV and avoid coverage of introitus/labia to minimize dermatitis
    - Small bowel contrast: may be useful to delineate small bowel
    - IV: generally not necessary. Only given when useful for nodal contouring. Assess risk for allergy/kidney injury.

    CT scan parameter: T9 to mid-femur
    Contouring

    - Targets: bilateral internal and external iliac nodal regions, vaginal cuff
    - OARs: small and large bowel, bladder, bone marrow, kidneys, external genitalia

    Prescription: 45–50.4 Gy in 1.8Gy fractions (if combined with IVRT 45Gy)
  - Intracavitary/interstitial brachytherapy [5, 6]

    MRI prior to brachytherapy for tumor geometry assessment

    General anesthesia

    Placement of applicator (interstitial/intracavitary) under image guidance (typically transrectal ultrasound)

    CT/MRI for treatment planning (MR preferred)

    Prescription: 4–5Gy x 5 fractions for total target EQD2 70–75Gy (medically inoperable 7–8.5Gy x 3–4 fractions with 1–2 insertions)
- Toxicity Management
  - Weekly CBCs with concurrent chemotherapy
  - Diarrhea: BRAT diet, anti-diarrheals, hydration/electrolyte repletion
  - Cystitis: interstitial cystitis diet, anti-inflammatories, rule out UTI
  - Perineal dermatitis: peribottle, cool compress, vaginal moisturizers, silver sulfasalazine for moist desquamation
  - Chronic bowel irritability: lactose-free diet, priobiotics (although weak evidence)
  - Radiation proctitis (rectal bleeding): fiber supplements, steroid suppositories, hyperbaric oxygen
  - Vaginal stenosis: start vaginal dilation 2–4 weeks post-treatment and continue until 6–12 months post-treatment. Vaginal moisturizers. Consider sexual health referral
- Follow-up
  - Every 3 months for the first 2 years, then every 6 months until year 5, then annually

Cervical Cancer

Clinical History and Diagnostic Evaluation

- Abnormal vaginal discharge/bleeding: (quality/timing/duration/extent, last gyn/PAP exam)
- Abdominopelvic symptoms: pain/discomfort, bowel or urinary changes
- Full GYN history: last GYN exam/PAP, history of HPV/vaccine, parity
- Imaging: MRI pelvis with/without contrast, PET
- GYN surgical oncology/Medical Oncology consultations

Adjuvant Therapy

- Intermediate risk (Sedlis criteria [8]): EBRT 45–50.4Gy

- High risk (Peters criteria [9]): EBRT 45–50.4Gy + concurrent cisplatin
- +vaginal margins: EBRT 45Gy + IVRT boost 15Gy/3f fractions.
- *mitigating pathologic and/or clinical features may impact decision-making regarding adjuvant therapy. Multidisciplinary discussion recommended.

Definitive Therapy

- IB2-IVa: definitive EBRT + brachytherapy boost with *concurrent chemotherapy
- *concurrent chemotherapy = cisplatin 40 mg/m2 x 6 doses
- Node negative: EBRT 45Gy
- Node positive: EBRT 45Gy + SIB (GTVn +0.5 cm) 56.25Gy
- Techniques [7, 10, 11]:
  - Simulation:

    Supine, Aquaplast mold, IV, oral, rectal, and vaginal contrast.

    Alpha cradle with arms above head if including the PA lymph nodes

    Isocenter: in center of pelvis
- As for endometrial cancer, we do not routinely utilize a full and empty bladder simulation and creation of an ITV
  - Contouring:

    Cover common, internal and external iliacs, obturator vessels, and presacral lymph nodes +0.7 cm expansion for nodal CTV (exclude bone and bowel)

    Cover inguinal nodes if lower 1/3 vaginal involvement

    Cover para-aortic nodes (up to renal vessels) if common iliac n+

    +0. 7 cm uniform expansion for nodal PTV

  Intact uterus:

    Contour uterus and cervix + any gross disease +2 cm expansion for primary PTV. Avoid including introitus/anal verge if feasible.

    Ensure PTV expansion extends to sidewall (bone) and thus includes parametria, but should not extend beyond sidewall

    Prioritize coverage of disease over OARs

  Postop:

    Similar to post-op endometrial contours with the inclusion of presacral nodes

  *Use IMRT to minimize bone marrow and GI toxicity

- Brachytherapy starts when optimal tumor geometry (generally after week 4 or 5)
- Selection of applicator based on disease extent on pre-brachytherapy MRI obtained as close to scheduled procedure as feasible
- Intracavitary (2 insertions, 1 week apart): 2 fx per week
- Interstitial (1 insertion, 1 wk. post EBRT) for interstitial-fx min 6 h apart
- 3D planning with MRI

- Volumes/target dose (EQD2) defined:
- GTV: all visible gross disease
- High Risk CTV: GTV + cervix—target dose = D90 85–95Gy
- Intermediate Risk CTV: HR CTV + 0.5 cm (excluding OARs)—target dose = D90–60–65Gy
- OARS: rectum (D90 < 70Gy), bladder (D90 < 85–90Gy), rectosigmoid (D90 < 70Gy), bowel (D90 < 60Gy)
- Toxicity Management
  - Similar to endometrial ca
  - Bone complications (insufficiency fractures, AVN):
    Ca/Vit D
    Pain control, early mobilization with physical therapy
    Bisphosphonates (or refer to Endocrinology)
    If immobilized: DVT prophylaxis
  - Ovarian transposition consideration prior to treatment (node neg); hormone replacement considered for young pts post-treatment
  - Hematologic: keep hgb >8
- Followup
  - Every 3mo for first 2 years with imaging (MR GYN and PET (until neg) then every 6mos until year 5 then annually.

Vulvar Cancer

Clinical history and diagnostic evaluation:

- Vulvar symptoms: pruritis/bleeding/mass; rule out multifocality
- History of HPV, lichen sclerosis, vulvar dysplasia, Paget's disease, smoking history, immune deficiency
- Imaging: MRI; PET
- Vulvar biopsy
- GYN Surgical Oncology and Medical Oncology consultation

Adjuvant therapy:

- High risk primary tumor features: +/close margins, deep invasion (>0.5 cm), tumor thickness > 0.5 cm: EBRT
- High risk nodal disease: ≥2LN + or ECE: EBRT [12]

Definitive therapy:

- Unresectable/Stage III/IVa: EBRT + *concurrent chemotherapy
- *cisplatin 40 mg/m2 weekly

Techniques [13]*:*

Simulation

- Supine, legs together or frog leg position, Alpha cradle, vaginal, rectal, IV, PO contrast, wire gross disease or scar post-op
- Bolus: only for frog leg position
- Place OSLDs at first fx to confirm adequate vulvar skin dose

Contouring

- Primary volume: gross tumor/bed + entire vulva, ensuring sufficient inferior margin (2 cm)
- Nodal volume: bilateral inguinal, internal, external, obturator, and iliac lymph nodes up to common iliac bifurcation
  Cover at least 2 cm above the highest node
  Ipsilateral nodal coverage can only be considered for well-lateralized, small tumors with documented ipsilateral drainage on SLND

Dosing

- Postop primary bed: negative margins: 50Gy in 2Gy fractions
  close margins: 54Gy in 2Gy fractions
  positive margins: 60Gy in 2Gy fractions
- Primary (unresectable/gross disease): 64Gy in 2 Gy fractions
- Clinically N0- 50Gy in 2Gy fractions
- Clinically N+ or ECE- 45Gy in 1.8Gy/60Gy in 2.4Gy fractions
- *minimize treatment interruptions with aggressive skin care and pain management
- *opportunity for adaptive therapy. Consider replan to reduce morbidity if substantial ontreatment tumor response

Toxicity management:

- Similar to endometrial
- Perineal dermatitis: peribottle, vulvar moisturizers, cool compress, cotton/loose undergarments, silver sulfasalazine for moist desquamation, oral/topical pain management as needed, rule out infection. Avoid astringents
- Lymphedema management: compression garments, massage, early physical therapy referral
- Hormone replacement therapy and/or Sexual Health referral for premenopausal women.

Followup

- Every 3mo for first 2 years with CT CAP then q6mo until year 5 then annually

Vaginal Cancer

Clinical history and diagnostic evaluation:

- Vaginal symptoms: bleeding/mass, urinary or bowel symptoms; rule out cervical primary
- History of HPV, smoking history, immune deficiency
- Imaging: MRI; PET
- Vaginal biopsy
- GYN Surgical Oncology and Medical Oncology consultation

Adjuvant therapy

- Close/positive margins or LN+: EBRT + concurrent chemotherapy +/– intravaginal brachytherapy boost (positive margins)

Definitive therapy

- Stage I: intravaginal brachytherapy (lesions <2 cm, thickness < 5 mm)
- Stage II–IVa: EBRT + concurrent chemotherapy + intracavitary/interstitial brachytherapy boost
- *concurrent chemotherapy = cisplatin 40 mg/m2 weekly

Techniques:

- Simulation:
  - Supine, Aquaplast immobilization, vaginal contrast with marker at introitus +/– anal verge. IV/Oral contrast may be considered.
- Contouring
  - Primary site + whole vagina + cervix with 1.5–2 cm margin = primary PTV
  - Nodal volumes include bilateral common iliac, internal, external iliac, presacral, obturator nodes and inguinal nodes (lower 1/3 lesions).
- Dosing
  - Close/positive margins: 54Gy in 1.8Gy
  - Clinically N0: 45Gy in 1.8Gy fractions
  - Clinically N+: 45Gy in 1.8Gy fractions with SIB to gross node/s + 0.5 cm to 56.25 Gy in 2.25Gy fractions
  - Interstitial/intravaginal boost: 4–5Gy in 5 fractions (EQD2 70–75Gy)
    Distal vaginal lesions favor 4Gy fractions
    For small Stage I lesions planned for brachytherapy alone: 40Gy in 8 fractions (EQD2 50–60Gy)

Toxicity Management

- Same for cervical/vulvar

Followup

- Every 3 months for the first 2 years with imaging, then q6mo until year 5, then annual

References

1. Pecorelli S. Revised FIGO staging for carcinoma of the vulva, cervix, and endometrium. Int J Gynaecol Obstet. 2009;105(2):103–4.
2. Eskander RN, et al. Pembrolizumab plus chemotherapy in advanced endometrial cancer. N Engl J Med. 2023;388(23):2159–70.
3. Mirza MR, et al. Dostarlimab for primary advanced or recurrent endometrial cancer. N Engl J Med. 2023;388(23):2145–58.
4. Schwarz JK, et al. Consensus statement for brachytherapy for the treatment of medically inoperable endometrial cancer. Brachytherapy. 2015;14(5):587–99.
5. Nag S, et al. The American Brachytherapy society recommendations for high-dose-rate brachytherapy for carcinoma of the endometrium. Int J Radiat Oncol Biol Phys. 2000;48(3):779–90.
6. Albuquerque K, et al. Compendium of fractionation choices for gynecologic HDR brachytherapy—an American Brachytherapy Society Task Group Report. Brachytherapy. 2019;18(4):429–36.
7. Small W Jr, et al. NRG Oncology/RTOG consensus guidelines for delineation of clinical target volume for intensity modulated pelvic radiation therapy in postoperative treatment of endometrial and cervical cancer: an update. Int J Radiat Oncol Biol Phys. 2021;109(2):413–24.
8. Sedlis A, et al. A randomized trial of pelvic radiation therapy versus no further therapy in selected patients with stage IB carcinoma of the cervix after radical hysterectomy and pelvic lymphadenectomy: a Gynecologic Oncology Group Study. Gynecol Oncol. 1999;73(2):177–83.
9. Peters WA 3rd, et al. Concurrent chemotherapy and pelvic radiation therapy compared with pelvic radiation therapy alone as adjuvant therapy after radical surgery in high-risk early-stage cancer of the cervix. J Clin Oncol. 2000;18(8):1606–13.
10. Viswanathan, A.N., B. Thomadsen, C. American Brachytherapy Society Cervical Cancer Recommendations, and S. American Brachytherapy. American Brachytherapy Society consensus guidelines for locally advanced carcinoma of the cervix. Part I: general principles. Brachytherapy. 2012;11(1):33–46.
11. Viswanathan AN, et al. American Brachytherapy Society consensus guidelines for locally advanced carcinoma of the cervix. Part II: high-dose-rate brachytherapy. Brachytherapy. 2012;11(1):47–52.
12. Oonk MHM, et al. Radiotherapy versus inguinofemoral lymphadenectomy as treatment for vulvar cancer patients with micrometastases in the sentinel node: results of GROINSS-V II. J Clin Oncol. 2021;39(32):3623–32.
13. Gaffney DK, et al. Consensus recommendations for radiation therapy contouring and treatment of vulvar carcinoma. Int J Radiat Oncol Biol Phys. 2016;95(4):1191–200.

10 Sarcoma

Jacob Y. Shin, Boris Mueller, and Kaled Alektiar

History and Workup

Essential components of the history and workup for soft tissue sarcoma include:

- Age
- Size
- Margin status (if resected)
- Grade of tumor
- Histology

Postoperative radiation therapy is indicated, in general, for deep, large tumors or those with positive margins. MSKCC Nomogram can be used to estimate local recurrence risk [1].

Imaging

- MRI: T1 POST to evaluate for enhancing mass, T2 for surrounding edema
- CT of the chest to evaluate for metastatic disease

Preoperative Treatment

If preoperative treatment is planned, the patient will need a referral to an oncological surgeon for an incisional biopsy.

J. Y. Shin (✉) · B. Mueller · K. Alektiar
Department of Radiation Oncology, Memorial Sloan Kettering Cancer Center, New York, NY, USA
e-mail: shinj2@mskcc.org; muellerb@mskcc.org; alektiak@mskcc.org

J. J. Cuaron, L. Z. Braunstein (eds.), *Radiation Oncology Clinical Fundamentals*,
https://doi.org/10.1007/978-3-031-77559-8_10

Preoperative treatment requires smaller radiotherapy fields and is associated with a lower risk of fibrosis and a higher risk of postoperative wound complications, especially in the lower extremities

DOSE:

- 50 Gy in 25 fractions, IMRT

SIMULATION:

- Positioning depends on location of primary; in the lower extremity, the treated leg will remain in neutral position and the unaffected leg will be manipulated outside of the treatment fields (usually akimbo).
- Immobilization typically combines alpha cradle and Aquaplast mold.
- No bolus

CONTOURING:

- GTV = tumor
- CTV: + 4 cm long, 1.0 radially
- PTV: +0.5 cm

IMAGING:

- Daily imaging (KV)

Post-Op Treatment

Postoperative treatment generally involves larger fields due to the need to cover the entire postoperative bed and margin. Postoperative treatment is associated with a higher risk of fibrosis and a lower risk of wound complications compared to preoperative treatment.

DOSE:

- 45 Gy with conedown to 63 Gy, IMRT

SIMULATION:

- Positioning depends on location of primary; in the lower extremity, the treated leg will remain in neutral position and the unaffected leg will be manipulated outside of the treatment fields (usually akimbo).
- Immobilization typically combines alpha cradle and Aquaplast mold.
- No bolus

CONTOURING:

- Contour pre-op GTV
- Contour tumor bed (hypodensity surrounding surgical clips)
- CTV45: expansion on tumor bed is 1 cm radially, 4 cm sup/inf excluding bone and external
- PTV45: CTV45 + 0.5 cm radially as long as daily kV imaging is performed (4500 cGy/25); do not Boolean with external; no bolus
- CTV63: expansion on tumor bed is 1 cm radially (4500 cGy + 1800 cGy/10 cone down)
- PTV63: CTV63 + 0.5 cm radially; do not Boolean with external; no bolus

Retroperitoneal Sarcoma

- Where vascular reconstruction is being considered:
  - Dose paint the posterior (dose painting 50.4 Gy /60.2 Gy in 28 fractions whole volume; 60.2 Gy to posterior structures excluding bowel).
- For other cases:
- SBRT 30 Gy in 5 fractions whole volume with field design, exclude contralateral kidney

CONTOURING:

- IMRT
  - Contour GTV
  - CTV: 1.5 cm uniformly from tumor
  - PTV: CTV + 0.5 cm uniformly
- SBRT
  - Contour GTV
  - CTV: 0.5 cm uniformly
  - PTV: CTV + 0.3 cm uniformly

Truncal Sarcoma (Chest Wall/Abdominal Wall)

DOSE:

- 45 Gy with conedown to 59.4 Gy, IMRT

CONTOURING:

- Contour pre-op GTV (using fused pre-op imaging)
- Contour tumor bed (hypodensity surrounding surgical clips)
- CTV45: expansion on tumor bed is 1cm radially, 2.5cm sup/inf excluding bone, external, or chest/abdominal cavity

- PTV45: CTV45 + 0.5cm uniform expansion as long as daily kV imaging is performed (4500cGy/25); do not Boolean with external; no bolus
- CTV59.4: tumor bed + 1cm uniform expansion (4500cGy/25 + 1440cGy/8 cone down)
- PTV59.4: CTV59.4 + 0.5cm uniform expansion; do not Boolean with external; no bolus

Head and Neck Sarcoma

DOSE:

- 180 × 35 = 6300 cGy

  CONTOURING:

- Contour tumor bed
- 1 cm from tumor bed to CTV all around
- 0.5 cm from CTV to PTV

Planning and Treatment Delivery

On Treatment Imaging

- IMRT: Daily KVs matched to bone with weekly CBCT
- SBRT: Daily KV and CBCT

On Treatment Management and Follow-Up Care

COMMON TOXICITIES:

- Management of Dermatitis: Emollients→mometasone→silvadene
- Early referral for therapy if suspicion of lymphedema

  FOLLOW–UP:

- At 6 weeks for toxicity check. Further follow-up at the discretion of the physician in conjunction with other providers.

References

1. Cahlon O, Brennan MF, Jia X, Qin LX, Singer S, Alektiar KM. A postoperative nomogram for local recurrence risk in extremity soft tissue sarcomas after limb-sparing surgery without adjuvant radiation. Ann Surg. 2012;255(2):343–7.

Further Reading

Alektiar KM, Brennan MF, Healey JH, Singer S. Impact of intensity-modulated radiation therapy on local control in primary soft-tissue sarcoma of the extremity. J Clin Oncol. 2008;26(20):3440–4. https://doi.org/10.1200/JCO.2008.16.6249.

Alektiar KM, Brennan MF, Singer S. Local control comparison of adjuvant brachytherapy to intensity-modulated radiotherapy in primary high-grade sarcoma of the extremity. Cancer. 2011;117(14):3229–34. https://doi.org/10.1002/cncr.25882.

Bishop AJ, Zagars GK, Torres KE, Hunt KK, Cormier JN, Feig BW, Guadagnolo BA. Combined modality management of retroperitoneal sarcomas: a single-institution series of 121 patients. Int J Radiat Oncol Biol Phys. 2015;93(1):158–65. https://doi.org/10.1016/j.ijrobp.2015.04.047.

Bonvalot S, Gronchi A, Le Pechoux C, et al. Preoperative radiotherapy plus surgery versus surgery alone for patients with primary retroperitoneal sarcoma (EORTC-62092: STRASS): a multicentre, open-label, randomised, phase 3 trial. Lancet Oncol. 2020;21(10):1366–77. https://doi.org/10.1016/S1470-2045(20)30446-0.

Chouliaras K, Senehi R, Ethun CG, et al. Role of radiation therapy for retroperitoneal sarcomas: an eight-institution study from the US Sarcoma Collaborative. J Surg Oncol. 2019;120(7):1227–34. https://doi.org/10.1002/jso.25694.

Diamantis A, Baloyiannis I, Magouliotis DE, et al. Perioperative radiotherapy versus surgery alone for retroperitoneal sarcomas: a systematic review and meta-analysis. Radiol Oncol. 2020;54(1):14–21. https://doi.org/10.2478/raon-2020-0012.

Folkert MR, Singer S, Brennan MF, et al. Comparison of local recurrence with conventional and intensity-modulated radiation therapy for primary soft-tissue sarcomas of the extremity. J Clin Oncol. 2014;32(29):3236–41. https://doi.org/10.1200/JCO.2013.53.9452.

Haas RLM, Bonvalot S, Miceli R, et al. Radiotherapy for retroperitoneal liposarcoma: a report from the Transatlantic Retroperitoneal Sarcoma Working Group. Cancer. 2019;125(8):1290–300. https://doi.org/10.1002/cncr.31927.

Kelly KJ, Yoon SS, Kuk D, et al. Comparison of perioperative radiation therapy and surgery versus surgery alone in 204 patients with primary retroperitoneal sarcoma: a retrospective 2-institution study. Ann Surg. 2015;262(1):156–62. https://doi.org/10.1097/SLA.0000000000001063.

Le Pechoux C, Musat E, Baey C, et al. Should adjuvant radiotherapy be administered in addition to front-line aggressive surgery (FAS) in patients with primary retroperitoneal sarcoma? Ann Oncol. 2013;24(3):832–7. https://doi.org/10.1093/annonc/mds516.

Pawlik TM, Pisters PW, Mikula L, et al. Long-term results of two prospective trials of preoperative external beam radiotherapy for localized intermediate- or high-grade retroperitoneal soft tissue sarcoma. Ann Surg Oncol. 2006;13(4):508–17. https://doi.org/10.1245/ASO.2006.05.035.

Pisters PW, Harrison LB, Leung DH, Woodruff JM, Casper ES, Brennan MF. Long-term results of a prospective randomized trial of adjuvant brachytherapy in soft tissue sarcoma. J Clin Oncol. 1996;14(3):859–68. https://doi.org/10.1200/JCO.1996.14.3.859.

Rosenberg SA, Tepper J, Glatstein E, et al. The treatment of soft-tissue sarcomas of the extremities: prospective randomized evaluations of (1) limb-sparing surgery plus radiation therapy compared with amputation and (2) the role of adjuvant chemotherapy. Ann Surg. 1982;196(3):305–15. https://doi.org/10.1097/00000658-198209000-00009.

Siegel RL, Giaquinto AN, Jemal A. Cancer statistics, 2024. CA Cancer J Clin. 2024;74(1):12–49. https://doi.org/10.3322/caac.21820.

Yang JC, Chang AE, Baker AR, et al. Randomized prospective study of the benefit of adjuvant radiation therapy in the treatment of soft tissue sarcomas of the extremity. J Clin Oncol. 1998;16(1):197–203. https://doi.org/10.1200/JCO.1998.16.1.197.

Hematological Malignancies

11

Carla Hajj, Brandon Imber, and Joachim Yahalom

History and Workup

Four major groups of diseases:

- Hodgkin lymphoma Diagnostic PET scan
  - B symptoms (drenching night sweats, weight loss>10% body weight within 6 months, and fever >38 °C)
  - Erythrocyte sedimentation rate (ESR)
  - Bone marrow biopsy (optional for early staged favorable risk)
- Non-Hodgkin lymphoma Diagnostic PET scan
  - Lactate Dehydrogenase (LDH)
  - Diagnostic PET scan
- Plasmacytoma/multiple myeloma
  - Protein electrophoresis (serum: SPEP and urine: UPEP)
  - Bone marrow biopsy
  - Skeletal survey
  - Diagnostic PET scan
  - Microglobulin level
- Leukemias

C. Hajj (✉) · B. Imber · J. Yahalom
Radiation Oncology Department, Memorial Sloan Kettering Cancer Center,
New York, NY, USA
e-mail: Hajjc@clevelandclinicabudhabi.ae; imberb@mskcc.org; yahalomj@mskcc.org

J. J. Cuaron, L. Z. Braunstein (eds.), *Radiation Oncology Clinical Fundamentals*,
https://doi.org/10.1007/978-3-031-77559-8_11

Hodgkin Lymphoma

Management

Early-Stage Favorable Hodgkin Lymphoma

Patients with early-stage favorable Hodgkin lymphoma are treated with 2 cycles of adriamycin, bleomycin, vinblastine, dacarbazine (ABVD) chemotherapy, followed by a restaging PET scan. Treatment response is assessed using the Deauville 5-point scale, where each fluorodeoxyglucose (FDG)-avid (or previously Fluorodeoxyglucose (FDG)-avid) lesions are rated independently:

1. No uptake or no residual uptake
2. Slight uptake, but equal to or below blood pool (mediastinum)
3. Uptake above mediastinal, but below or equal to uptake in the liver
4. Uptake slightly to moderately higher than liver
5. Markedly increased uptake or any new lesion (on response evaluation)

Patients with a Deauville score ranging from 1–4 after 2 cycles of ABVD are treated with involved site radiation treatment (ISRT) to 20Gy in 2Gy per fraction. Patients with a Deauville score of 5 are considered to have refractory disease and, after biopsy confirmation, are treated with ifosfamide, carboplatin, etoposide (ICE) chemotherapy and radiation treatment to the initial sites of bulky disease to achieve a complete response, followed by consideration of an autologous stem cell transplant.

Early-Stage Unfavorable Hodgkin Lymphoma

Patients with early-stage unfavorable Hodgkin lymphoma are treated with 4 cycles of ABVD, followed by a restaging PET scan. Response to chemotherapy is also assessed using the Deauville 5-point score. Patients with a Deauville score of 1–3 can receive an additional 2 cycles of ABVD, followed by ISRT to 30Gy in 2Gy per fraction. Patients with a Deauville score of 4 will receive 2 more cycles of ABVD, followed by a restaging PET scan. Patients with a Deauville score of 5 will undergo a biopsy, and if chemorefractory disease is confirmed, they would be considered for stem cell transplant.

Advanced-Stage Hodgkin Lymphoma

Patients with stage III or IV disease are treated with 6 cycles of ABVD, followed by a restaging PET scan. ISRT to 30Gy is indicated in patients with bulky sites at presentation and those with a partial response after restaging PET scan.

Nodular Lymphocyte Predominant Hodgkin Lymphoma

Those patients are treated with ISRT to 30Gy in 2Gy per fraction as a single modality treatment. Systemic therapy is indicated in patients who achieve a partial response after ISRT.

Simulation

Response to chemotherapy should be coordinated with simulation.

- PET/CT simulation in the treatment position
  - The PET/CT scan will serve to assess response to systemic therapy and to plan the radiation treatment.
- Immobilization devices, contrast, and motion management techniques are a function of the treated sites.
  - Neck: Arms down in a 5-point mask, 100 cc of IV iodine contrast.
  - Chest: Arms up in an alpha cradle, 100 cc of IV iodine contrast. Simulation and treatment are done with deep inspiration breath hold (DIBH), which allows for reduction of mediastinal volume and expansion of lung volume.
- The isocenter is placed in the center of the CTV.

Contouring

We follow the involved site radiation therapy (ISRT) guidelines as defined by the International Lymphoma Radiation Oncology Group (ILROG) [1].

Diffuse Large B-Cell Lymphoma (DLBCL)

Management

Early-Stage DLBCL

Patients with early-stage DLBCL are treated with 3 cycles of rituximab, cyclophosphamide, doxorubicin, vincristine, prednisone (R-CHOP) chemotherapy followed by ISRT. The dose of radiation treatment depends on the response to systemic therapy and initial disease presentation. Patients in complete response after R-CHOP are treated with 30Gy in 2Gy per fraction ISRT if no initial bulky disease, and 36Gy in 2Gy per fraction in case of bulky disease at presentation. Patients with a partial response to 3 cycles of R-CHOP will receive an additional 3 cycles of R-CHOP followed by 40Gy in 2Gy per fraction consolidation RT in case of partial response and 46Gy in 2Gy per fraction in case of disease progression.

Advance-Stage DLBCL

Patients with early-stage DLBCL are treated with 6 cycles of R-CHOP, followed by ISRT to 36Gy in 2Gy per fraction to initially bulky sites of disease.

Double-Hit DLBCL (All Stages)

Those patients are treated with either 6 cycles of R-CHOP followed by 30Gy in 2Gy per fraction ISRT versus DA-R-EPOCH dose-adjusted Rituximab, Etoposide, Prednisone, Vincristine (Oncovin), Cyclophosphamide, Doxorubicin hydrochloride (Hydroxydaunorubicin) chemotherapy.

Simulation

Same principles as for Hodgkin lymphoma patients.

Contouring

We follow the ISRT guidelines as defined by the International Lymphoma Radiation Oncology Group (ILROG) [2].

Follicular Lymphoma (FL)/Non-gastric Marginal Zone Lymphoma (MZL)

Management

Early-Stage

Patients with early-stage FL or MZL are treated with ISRT to 24Gy in 2Gy per fraction per standard of care. In select cases (size<6 cm, SUV<10), an adapted approach can also be used, where patients are treated to 4Gy either in a single fraction (4Gy×1 Big Boom) or two fractions (2Gy×2 Boom Boom). In case of partial response to 4Gy on restaging PET scan done 8 weeks post-radiation therapy, a definitive dose to a total of 24Gy is offered.

Advanced-Stage

Patients with advanced FL or MZL can be observed or treated with Rituximab alone or with R-CHOP. RT to 4Gy either in a single fraction (4Gy×1 Big Boom) or two fractions (2Gy×2 Boom Boom) can be used for palliation.

Simulation

Same principles as for Hodgkin lymphoma patients.

Contouring

We follow the ISRT guidelines as defined by the International Lymphoma Radiation Oncology Group (ILROG) [2].

Common Lymphoma Treatment Regimens

In Table 11.1, we summarize the most used doses and fractionation schemes to treat hematologic malignancies, in addition to the short-course regimens proposed by the ILROG for radiation therapy of hematological malignancies during the COVID-19 pandemic [3].

On Treatment Management and Follow-Up Care

Common Toxicities

Radiation-induced toxicities depend on the irradiated organ and surrounding organs at risk. We will address in this section how we manage commonly encountered toxicities.

Table 11.1 The most used doses and fractionation schemes to treat hematologic malignancies

DIAGNOSIS	DOSE	IMAGING
Hodgkin lymphoma—Favorable, chemosensitive (standard)	200 cGy × 10	2DKV daily, CBCT weekly
Hodgkin lymphoma—Favorable, chemosensitive (short course)	300 × 6	2DKV daily, CBCT weekly
Hodgkin lymphoma—Unfavorable, chemosensitive OR NLPHL RT alone (standard)	200 × 15	2DKV daily, CBCT weekly
Hodgkin lymphoma—Unfavorable, chemosensitive OR NLPHL RT alone (short course)	300 × 9	2DKV daily, CBCT weekly
Hodgkin lymphoma—Chemorefractory	200 × 20 OR 300 × 12	2DKV daily, CBCT weekly
Hodgkin lymphoma—Salvage pre-transplant	150 × 20	2DKV daily, CBCT weekly
Non-Hodgkin lymphoma—Chemosensitive long course	200 × 15	2DKV daily, CBCT weekly
Non-Hodgkin lymphoma—Chemosensitive short course	300 × 9 (mediastinum) OR 500 × 5 (non-mediastinum)	2DKV daily, CBCT weekly
Non-Hodgkin Lymphoma—chemorefractory OR local aggressive for RT alone (standard)	200 × 23	2DKV daily, CBCT weekly
Non-Hodgkin lymphoma—Chemorefractory OR local aggressive for RT alone (short course)	300 × 12	2DKV daily, CBCT weekly
Non-Hodgkin lymphoma—Chemorefractory OR local aggressive For RT alone	500 × 6	2DKV daily, CBCT weekly
Limited stage indolent	200 × 12	2DKV daily, CBCT weekly
Limited stage indolent (boom)	400 × 1	2DKV daily, CBCT weekly

- Cough: First-line treatment of cough is Guaifenesin and codeine, followed by benzonatate pearls, and then homatropine/hydrocodone.
- Esophagitis: We start by recommending diet modification, then prescribe proton pump inhibitors, sucralfate, and then transition to opiates. Hydration and/or admission are recommended on an as-needed basis.
- Dermatitis: Emollients, Mometasone cream, and silver sulfadiazine are prescribed depending on the grade of radiation dermatitis.

Follow-Up Care

- All patients are seen at 6 weeks for a toxicity check with a repeat CT vs. PET/CT scan for response assessment. Restaging imaging needs to be coordinated with medical oncology.
- Further follow-up is indicated at the discretion of the treating physician.

References

1. Specht L, et al. Modern radiation therapy for Hodgkin lymphoma: field and dose guidelines from the international lymphoma radiation oncology group (ILROG). Int J Radiat Oncol Biol Phys. 2014;89(4):854–62.
2. Illidge T, et al. Modern radiation therapy for nodal non- Hodgkin lymphoma-target definition and dose guidelines from the International Lymphoma Radiation Oncology Group. Int J Radiat Oncol Biol Phys. 2014;89(1):49–58.
3. Yahalom J, et al. ILROG emergency guidelines for radiation therapy of hematological malignancies during the COVID-19 pandemic. Blood. 2020;135(21):1829–32.

Non-Spine Bone Metastases and Extracranial Soft Tissue

12

David Guttmann, Amy Xu, Daniel Gomez, and Jonathan Yang

Introduction

Treatment of metastatic disease accounts for a large proportion of clinical practice in radiation oncology. Many classic techniques of palliative radiotherapy remain unchanged after decades of use and are familiar to practicing radiation oncologists. An important exception, however, is the emerging use of highly conformal techniques such as Stereotactic body radiotherapy (SBRT) in the treatment of metastatic disease.

SBRT in the treatment of lung, liver, brain, and spinal metastases is well-described in the literature and is addressed in other chapters of this textbook. However, SBRT is also increasingly utilized in the management of non-spine osseous and extracranial soft tissue metastases [1]. While there is still ongoing controversy regarding which patients remain appropriate for this treatment, clinical presentations of oligometastatic disease, reirradiation after local progression, and radioresistant histologies are several common instances where SBRT for non-spine osseous and soft tissue lesions is being considered in the metastatic setting.

Much of the data on SBRT for non-spine extracranial metastases is formed by retrospective evidence, and in this context, consensus opinion and practice patterns are not yet standardized. Consequently, the specifics of simulation, contouring, planning, and treatment delivery described here should serve as a starting point for a description of the use of SBRT in management of: (a) non-spine bone and (b) non-bone extracranial metastatic disease. These techniques may only be appropriate in select circumstances and are often utilized within the context of a clinical trial.

D. Guttmann (✉) · A. Xu · D. Gomez
Department of Radiation Oncology, Memorial Sloan Kettering Cancer Center, New York, NY, USA

J. Yang
Department of Radiation Oncology, NYU School of Medicine, New York, NY, USA

J. J. Cuaron, L. Z. Braunstein (eds.), *Radiation Oncology Clinical Fundamentals*,
https://doi.org/10.1007/978-3-031-77559-8_12

It also must be emphasized that appropriate management of metastatic disease is truly a multidisciplinary effort involving radiation oncologists, medical oncologists, orthopedic surgeons, interventional radiology, pain management, and rehabilitation medicine, among other specialties. The focus here will be to highlight technical considerations for the radiation oncologist planning SBRT for non-spine extracranial metastases.

History and Workup

History and workup are critical to determining whether treatment is being delivered with palliative or ablative intent. A comprehensive history should elicit the patient's symptoms (intensity, onset, quality, exacerbating factors) and performance status (Karnofsky Performance Status or Eastern Cooperative Oncology Group (ECOG)). We also recommend discussing the patient's overall prognosis and goals of care with the patient, their primary medical oncologist, and supportive care specialists. Validated prognostic models may be helpful in assessing the appropriateness of treatment [2, 3]. Disease-specific considerations, such as intrinsic radiosensitivity and systemic therapy options, are also important in determining the appropriate course of metastasis-directed therapy.

Palliative radiation is an effective tool in alleviating symptoms from non-spine bone metastases and extracranial soft tissues, such as pain, obstruction, or bleeding. For bone lesions, it is important to assess for fracture risk using one of several available nomograms/algorithms (e.g., Mirels Criteria) [4] and differentiate between biologic and mechanical pain. Consider consultation with orthopedic surgery and/or interventional radiology for Mirel score 8+ and mechanical symptoms, especially for weight-bearing bones (peri-trochanteric, femur, tibia). Bisphosphonates can also be considered to reduce the risk of fracture. Complex clinical scenarios, including recurrence after initial local therapy or impending pathologic fracture, may benefit from multidisciplinary discussion [5].

For patients with limited ("oligo") sites of metastatic disease, emerging data suggest that ablative radiation doses may improve overall survival [6, 7]. Radiation administered with the intent of improving systemic disease progression should be designed with an appropriate biologic equivalent dose, such as what has been described in national oligometastatic trials [8]. As the role of ablative therapies for oligometastatic disease is under active investigation, every effort should be made to deliver such treatment on a clinical protocol, with appropriate referral to specialized centers for technically challenging treatments.

Imaging

We strongly recommend MRI and/or PET to assist in target delineation, particularly when utilizing ablative doses, as these modalities often reveal larger extents of disease spread than would be predicted on CT imaging alone. Pre-op and pre-chemo imaging can also be useful for delineating areas of microscopic spread.

Simulation

Immobilization should take into account tight planning target volume (PTV) margins and compatibility with image guidance. Oral contrast should be considered for lesions near GI luminal organs (barium for esophageal delineation, omnipaque for lower GI tract). For nodal targets and lesions near the brachial plexus, IV contrast may also be helpful. However, keep in mind that many metastatic patients may have limited kidney function due to medical comorbidities or toxicities from other systemic therapies. Thus, careful attention is warranted to consider the risk/benefit ratio of any contrast administration.

Contouring

Treatment of Intact Metastatic Lesions

Accurate target delineation is critical to maximize the chance of tumor control while minimizing risks of toxicity or local tumor progression, both of which may pose substantial cost to a patient under treatment for metastatic disease. ICRU conventions of gross tumor volume (GTV), clinical target volume (CTV), and planning target volume (PTV) apply in the treatment of metastatic targets in the same manner as in the definitive setting. Here, we will discuss how each are defined in the context of SBRT for non-spine bone and extracranial soft tissue metastases.

The GTV is often apparent on the CT imaging obtained during simulation. When considering osseous targets, lytic lesions are visible on CT as radiolucencies in the surrounding bone and blastic lesions as osseous radio-densities. Metastatic soft tissue lesions are often apparent on CT as aberrant or asymmetric soft tissue and may show contrast enhancement.

An important caveat here, however, is that while the CT simulation may serve as a starting point for contouring, CT alone can both under-estimate or overestimate the full extent of the viable tumor. Furthermore, some osseous and soft lesions will remain completely occult on CT. For these reasons, additional imaging, notably MRI or PET, can complement the CT simulation and improve accuracy in GTV delineation. While obtaining imaging beyond CT scans is not a requirement for all cases, all available diagnostic imaging should be incorporated into treatment planning. Obtaining additional dedicated MRI and PET/CT scans specifically for SBRT radiation planning may be warranted in cases where there is difficulty in appreciating the tumor extent on CT or when severely dose-limiting organs at risk (OARs) lay in close proximity to the treatment volume. These considerations may become even more important in the setting of reirradiation.

CTV delineation is accomplished by a uniform expansion off of the GTV, which can then be cropped from anatomic barriers to spread. Such barriers may include bone/soft tissue interfaces or neighboring organs in cases where a clear tissue plane can be visualized. However, certain metastatic lesions will cross tissue planes to invade neighboring tissues and so incorporating these into the CTV may sometimes be appropriate. For example, cropping at CTV at a bone/soft tissue interface would be inappropriate when there is concern for extraosseous tumor extension into the surrounding muscle.

There are no high-level data governing the optimal extent of GTV to CTV expansion, although consensus agreements indicate that 5-10 mm may be appropriate [9]. The exact extent of expansion will depend on the clinical context, including the patient's overall performance status, intent of treatment, neighboring OARs, field size, and prior radiation near or within the radiation field. Registering an MRI or PET to the simulation images may allow for a smaller GTV to CTV expansion by improving delineation of the tumor/normal tissue interface [10].

The use of an ITV (internal tumor volume) as per routine practice in cases of internal organ motion can be considered on a case by case basis and may be appropriate in the treatment of non-spine bone metastases with SBRT. In general, when radiation doses higher than standard palliative regimens are given, a 4D scan should be performed for tumors in the thorax and upper-mid abdomen. This paradigm may apply to the treatment of rib metastases, for example, and a 4D scan should be obtained for high doses to metastatic retroperitoneal lymph nodes and adrenal gland lesions. Various strategies exist to account for organ motion, including gated treatment, breath hold, or abdominal compression. Dedicated chapters on management of lung and liver metastases cover the discussion about management of organ motion in more detail.

Lastly, CTV to PTV expansion accounts for setup uncertainty and must factor in the immobilization, technical capabilities, and reliability of patient setup at the treating facility. Often 3-5 mm margins are appropriate in the case of SBRT for non-spine bone metastases, contingent upon the IGRT modality used.

Special Considerations in the Case of Postoperative and Preoperative Treatment

Occasionally, postoperative SBRT may be considered in the setting of treatment after surgical stabilization with an incomplete resection, particularly in the setting of radio-resistant histologies or when clinical factors dictate that treatment be completed expeditiously. Any available relevant preoperative and postoperative imaging should be registered with the planning simulation to ensure preoperative tumor extent is fully encompassed in the treatment. A generous CTV margin of at least 5-10 mm, but often including any potential area of tumor contamination during surgery, including the entire surgical hardware, may be appropriate [11].

Pre-operative SBRT for high-risk metastatic lesions prior to a planned surgical stabilization is an area of emerging interest. There is little evidence to inform this treatment paradigm, and ideally such a practice should be performed in the context of a clinical trial.

Planning and Treatment Delivery

The optimal dose of radiation for appropriate palliation of non-spine bone metastases in the context of conventional radiation has been debated for decades. There are by comparison far fewer high-level data describing dose-prescription for SBRT for non-spine palliative radiation. Currently employed dose prescriptions are often a reflection of consensus opinion rather than high-level evidence.

Most common palliative SBRT regimens rely on 1–5 fraction-dose prescriptions. The choice among these regimens must account for goals of treatment, patient clinical characteristics, radiation sensitivity of the tumor, the multidisciplinary management of the patient, and neighboring OARs. Among 5 fraction conformal regimens, 25–30 Gy in 5 fractions is an often safe and well-tolerated regimen that can provide durable palliation, although aside from very radiosensitive histologies, it may not provide long-term local control. Further escalation to 35–40 Gy in 5 fractions with the goal of tumor ablation is also reasonable with appropriate planning techniques and IGRT if, for dosimetric reasons, an ablative 5-fraction regimen is preferred [7]. For 3 fraction regimens, 27–30 Gy in 3 fractions can also present a reasonable option, with the caveat that 27 Gy in 3 fractions has been associated with slightly worse local control outcomes compared to higher biologically effective doses [12, 13].

Single-fraction SBRT for management of non-spine bone metastases is appealing due to patient convenience and emerging evidence that single fraction SBRT may lead to improved outcomes in the right setting. Dose prescriptions for single fraction RT vary widely. 12–16 Gy × 1 has been demonstrated to be a safe and effective regimen for palliation in non-spine bone metastases [14]. Doses as high as 24 Gy × 1 have been shown to be safe and associated with improved outcomes compared to multi-fraction SBRT in terms of local and even distant metastatic control [12]. In practice, until further data emerges regarding the use of single fraction SBRT for non-spine bone metastases, it is preferable to reserve ablative single fraction RT for small lesions in non-weight-bearing structures remote from OARs.

Further nuance in radiation dosing can be considered with the use of simultaneous integrated boost dosing (SIB, or "dose-painting"), in which select regions of the total treatment volume—often the GTV or a central core of the treatment volume remote from OARs—are taken to a higher prescription dose. This can be an effective strategy to more safely dose escalate in regions adjacent to dose-limited OARs when treating with ablative dose RT [15].

On Treatment Management and Follow-Up Care

The presentation of toxicities from SBRT for non-spine bone metastases is highly variable depending on the treatment location, size, and dose delivered. Management here relies on the basic principles of symptomatic care for acute radiation side effects. A special consideration regarding the acute effects of SBRT concerns their time course relative to more protracted treatments. In some situations, the peak period of side effects may occur 1–2 weeks or longer after the completion of radiation. Patients should be counseled about this expectation, and it is important that lines of support are open to patients during this period to ensure acute effects are managed appropriately.

Pain flare is one noteworthy acute side effect after SBRT or even conventional RT for metastatic lesions. Pain flare presents as an acute inflammatory reaction to even a single dose of radiation that can result in mild to severe pain. There is evidence supporting prophylactic administration of dexamethasone in an effort to mitigate this [16]. Given that pain flare occurs in roughly 25–30% of cases, according to this study, routine use of prophylactic glucocorticoids may represent overtreatment in many cases. Therefore, it is often reasonable to advise patients on the risk of pain flare and help manage acute pain if and when it arises through either non-steroidal anti-inflammatories if medically appropriate, opioid or non-opioid analgesics, or steroidal agents.

References

1. Gillespie EF, Lapen K, Wang DG, et al. Replacing 30 Gy in 10 fractions with stereotactic body radiation therapy for bone metastases: a large multi-site single institution experience 2016-2018. Clin Transl Radiat Oncol. 2020;25:75–80.
2. Chow E, Fung K, Panzarella T, Bezjak A, Danjoux C, Tannock I. A predictive model for survival in metastatic cancer patients attending an outpatient palliative radiotherapy clinic. Int J Radiat Oncol Biol Phys. 2002;53:1291–302.
3. Krishnan MS, Epstein-Peterson Z, Chen Y-H, Tseng YD, Wright AA, Temel JS, Catalano P, Balboni TA. Predicting life expectancy in patients with metastatic cancer receiving palliative radiotherapy: the TEACHH model. Cancer. 2014;120:134–41.
4. Mirels H. Metastatic disease in long bones. A proposed scoring system for diagnosing impending pathologic fractures. Clin Orthop. 1989;(249):256–64.
5. Gillespie EF, Mathis NJ, Vaynrub M, et al. Multidisciplinary treatment of non-spine bone metastases: results of a modified Delphi consensus process. Clin Transl Radiat Oncol. 2022;35:76–83.
6. Gomez DR, Tang C, Zhang J, et al. Local consolidative therapy vs. maintenance therapy or observation for patients with oligometastatic non-small-cell lung cancer: long-term results of a multi-institutional, phase II, randomized study. J Clin Oncol Off J Am Soc Clin Oncol. 2019;37:1558–65.
7. Palma DA, Olson R, Harrow S, et al. Stereotactic ablative radiotherapy for the comprehensive treatment of oligometastatic cancers: long-term results of the SABR-COMET phase II randomized trial. J Clin Oncol Off J Am Soc Clin Oncol. 2020;38:2830–8.
8. Chmura S, Winter KA, Robinson C, et al. Evaluation of safety of stereotactic body radiotherapy for the treatment of patients with multiple metastases: findings from the NRG-BR001 phase 1 trial. JAMA Oncol. 2021;7:845–52.
9. Nguyen TK, Chin L, Sahgal A, et al. International multi-institutional patterns of contouring practice and clinical target volume recommendations for stereotactic body radiation therapy for non-spine bone metastases. Int J Radiat Oncol Biol Phys. 2022;112:351–60.
10. Nguyen TK, Sahgal A, Dagan R, et al. Stereotactic body radiation therapy for nonspine bone metastases: international practice patterns to guide treatment planning. Pract Radiat Oncol. 2020;10:e452–60.

11. Rosen DB, Haseltine JM, Bartelstein M, et al. Should postoperative radiation for long bone metastases cover part or all of the orthopedic hardware? Results of a large retrospective analysis. Adv Radiat Oncol. 2021;6:100756.
12. Zelefsky MJ, Yamada Y, Greco C, et al. Phase 3 multi-center, prospective, randomized trial comparing single-dose 24 Gy radiation therapy to a 3-fraction SBRT regimen in the treatment of oligometastatic cancer. Int J Radiat Oncol Biol Phys. 2021;110:672–9.
13. Ost P, Reynders D, Decaestecker K, et al. Surveillance or metastasis-directed therapy for oligometastatic prostate cancer recurrence: a prospective, randomized, multicenter phase II trial. J Clin Oncol Off J Am Soc Clin Oncol. 2018;36:446–53.
14. Nguyen Q-N, Chun SG, Chow E, et al. Single-fraction stereotactic vs conventional multifraction radiotherapy for pain relief in patients with predominantly nonspine bone metastases: a randomized phase 2 trial. JAMA Oncol. 2019;5:872–8.
15. Reyngold M, Parikh P, Crane CH. Ablative radiation therapy for locally advanced pancreatic cancer: techniques and results. Radiat Oncol Lond Engl. 2019;14:95.
16. Chow E, Meyer RM, Ding K, et al. Dexamethasone in the prophylaxis of radiation-induced pain flare after palliative radiotherapy for bone metastases: a double-blind, randomised placebo-controlled, phase 3 trial. Lancet Oncol. 2015;16:1463–72.

Index

J. J. Cuaron, L. Z. Braunstein (eds.), *Radiation Oncology Clinical Fundamentals*,
https://doi.org/10.1007/978-3-031-77559-8

MIX
Papier aus verantwortungsvollen Quellen
Paper from responsible sources
FSC® C105338

If you have any concerns about our products,
you can contact us on
ProductSafety@springernature.com

In case Publisher is established outside the EU,
the EU authorized representative is:
Springer Nature Customer Service Center GmbH
Europaplatz 3, 69115 Heidelberg, Germany

Printed by Libri Plureos GmbH
in Hamburg, Germany